PHYSIOLOGY - LABORATORY AND CLINICAL RESEARCH

REGULATION OF FATIGUE IN EXERCISE

PHYSIOLOGY - LABORATORY AND CLINICAL RESEARCH

SPORTS AND ATHLETICS PREPARATION, PERFORMANCE, AND PSYCHOLOGY

Additional books in this series can be found on Nova's website under the Series tab.

Additional E-books in this series can be found on Nova's website under the E-books tab.

PHYSIOLOGY - LABORATORY AND CLINICAL RESEARCH

REGULATION OF FATIGUE IN EXERCISE

FRANK E. MARINO
EDITOR

Nova Science Publishers, Inc.
New York

For permission to use material from this book please contact us:
Telephone 631-231-7269; Fax 631-231-8175
Web Site: http://www.novapublishers.com

LIBRARY OF CONGRESS CATALOGING-IN-PUBLICATION DATA

Regulation of fatigue in exercise / editors, Frank E. Marino.
p. cm. -- (Physiology - laboratory and clinical research)
Includes bibliographical references and index.
ISBN 978-1-61209-334-5 (hardcover : alk. paper)
1. Fatigue. 2. Exercise. 3. Health. 4. Stress (Physiology) 5. Exercise--Physiological aspects. 6. Sports--Physiological aspects. I. Marino, Frank E.
RA781.R33 2011
613--dc22

2011003737

Published by Nova Science Publishers, Inc. † New York

CONTENTS

PREFACE

The chapters contained within this edited volume are the result of presentations delivered at a meeting on the *Future of Fatigue in Exercise* July 19-21, 2009. The purpose of the meeting was to bring to the forefront new ideas about fatigue in exercise which have been proposed over the last 15 years or so. Much of the controversy in this area of research has stemmed from the insightful "unpacking" of the interpretations provided by proponents of the classical view that the limitations of human physical performance are determined primarily by the limitations of the circulatory system. One might argue that this view and understanding has stood the test of time and thus is unshakable in its abilities to predict human physical performance. However, it is noteworthy that the philosopher Karl Popper suggested that every idea might someday fall to the ground.

More important than Popper's assertion is the most sacred of tenets of scientific inquiry; that of refutation. The consequence of all scientific inquiry is that new models come to light which might better explain a wide range of phenomena. To this end, the chapters contained in this volume are intended to provide the reader with some alternative explanations for existing data and a way forward for those wanting to continue unraveling the causes of fatigue under various exercise conditions. If, by the reading this book the reader is not enticed to challenge or argue with the authors then the book will have missed an opportunity and not served its greater purpose. In saying this, it is worthwhile reiterating the wise words of renowned paleoanthropologists Johanson and Shreeve [1], "As scientists, our first responsibility is to squeeze the last drop of information out of every bit of evidence we have in hand. But we must also be willing to take the next step, and build from that information theories that will be ready when the next discovery comes along to test their strength. That's what doing science means…The point is not to be right. The point is to make progress. And you cannot make progress if you are afraid to be wrong." (p. 131). It is with this sense of adventure and willingness that the authors of the chapters in this book have undertaken their writing task.

[1] Johanson D, Shreeve J. Lucy's child: The discovery of a human ancestor. London: Viking; 1989.

In: Regulation of Fatigue in Exercise
Editor: Frank E. Marino
ISBN 978-1-61209-334-5

Chapter 1

THE CENTRAL GOVERNOR MODEL AND FATIGUE DURING EXERCISE

Timothy David Noakes *
UCT/MRC Research Unit for Exercise Science and Sports Medicine,
Department of Human Biology, University of Cape Town and Sports Science
Institute of South Africa, Boundary Road, Newlands, 7700, South Africa

ABSTRACT

In 1923 Nobel Laureate A.V. Hill proposed that maximal exercise performance is limited by the development of ischaemia of the heart leading to anaerobiosis in the exercising skeletal muscles. This anaerobiosis prevented the oxidative removal of the lactic acid that Hill believed induced skeletal muscle contraction. As a result, skeletal muscle relaxation was inhibited, impairing exercise performance and inducing fatigue. This theory has dominated teaching and research in the exercise sciences for the past 80 years. But the problem with the model is that there is little biological evidence that it is correct and much that disproves it. For example there is no evidence that skeletal muscles become "anaerobic" during exercise or that the accumulation of lactic acid impairs skeletal muscle function. Further this model of exercise performance is unable to explain at least 6 common phenomena including (i) differential pacing strategies for different exercise durations; (ii) the end spurt in most forms of competitive sport; the presence of fatigue even though (iii) homeostasis is maintained and (iv) fewer than 100% of the muscle fibers in the active limbs have been activated; (v) the ability of certain drugs and other interventions to enhance exercise performance even though they act exclusively on the brain; and (vi) the finding that the Rating of Perceived Exertion (RPE) is a function of the relative exercise duration rather than the exercise intensity. More importantly, the cardinal weakness of this model is that it is "brainless". It allows no role for the brain in the regulation of exercise performance. In this chapter I present the evidence that an alternate model of exercise performance, the Central Governor Model, is better able to explain all these phenomena. The CGM views exercise as a behaviour that is regulated in

* Tel: +2721 6502459; E-mail: timothy.noakes@uct.ac.za; noakes@iafrica.com

anticipation by complex intelligent systems in the brain, the function of which are to ensure that whole body homoeostasis is protected under all conditions. According to this complex model fatigue is purely an emotion, the function of which is to insure that exercise terminates before there is a catastrophic biological failure. The complexity of this regulation cannot be appreciated by those who study the body as if it is a collection of disconnected components, as has become the usual practice in the modern exercise sciences.

INTRODUCTION

My early career in the medical sciences was strongly influenced by Prof Christiaan Barnard who on the night of the 3rd December 1967, performed the world's first successful human heart transplant in my hometown. As a direct result, three months later whilst completing a student exchange program in Los Angeles, California, I decided to study Medicine at the University of Cape Town. After completing my training and my internship, I chose to complete an MD degree for which I studied, amongst other topics, the function of the heart using an isolated, perfused, pumping rat heart model. I wished to understand the nature of the factors that determine the heart's ability to produce a maximum cardiac output. Since a large focus of my subsequent career has been to challenge the theory that the cardiac output is the principal regulator of human exercise performance [1], only now do I appreciate the irony of that choice.

For five years I worked in Professor Lionel Opie's laboratory that was established at the University of Cape Town to study cardiac metabolism as a result of Professor Barnard's innovation. Perhaps my subsequent career was influenced by Professor Barnard's statement that: "Most of us think along straight lines, like a bus or a train or a tram. If the destination isn't up on the board, few of us would know where we are going - and this applies even to scientific researchers who should know better. We tend to let tradition lead us by the nose. It takes an effort of will to break out of the mould" [2] (p. 56).

During this research I discovered that an important factor determining the heart's capacity to produce a maximum cardiac output was the nature of the fuels and hormones supplied to it. Only when provided with glucose, insulin and adrenaline did the heart produce its highest cardiac output [3]. Importantly these chemicals maximized myocardial contractility [4], which is best understood as the capacity of each individual actin and myosin crossbridge to produce force during myocardial contraction; the greater the force produced by each cross-bridge, the higher the contractility. Looking back in hindsight at that work 30 years later, I now conclude that even though it lacks a brain to control it, the isolated working heart paces itself during these experiments so that it does not fail catastrophically. Instead it always functions with reserve but this reserve is minimized in hearts perfused with glucose, insulin and adrenaline. I learned also that the heart maximized its stroke volume and hence the cardiac output, through quite large changes in myocardial contractility. Subsequently we showed that physical training altered the extent of certain phosphorylation processes on the regulatory myosin light chains and that these changes might explain training-induced changes in myocardial contractility and hence in cardiac function [5].

Perhaps the single most important physiological principle I learned during that time was contained in Table 10.1 on page 162 of the 1977 version of the classic textbook of the time, *Physiology of the Heart,* written by Professor Arnold Katz [6] of New York. That table compared the mechanisms by which the heart and skeletal muscles increase their force production. It explains that skeletal muscle increases its force production almost entirely by increasing the number of motor units (and hence muscle fibers and cross-bridges) that are active (recruited) in the exercising muscles. Katz proposes the still common belief that skeletal muscle fibers have only a very limited capacity to increase their inherent contractility.

In contrast, because all its fibers contract with each beat, the heart cannot increase its force production through an increased muscle fiber recruitment. Instead this increase can occur only as a result of maximizing (i) the number of actin and myosin cross bridges formed during contraction (the Frank-Starling effect) and (ii) the contractility of each cross-bridge. The strange paradox is that those cardiologists who have little direct contact with the exercise sciences, have always taught that skeletal muscle increases its contractile force by recruiting more motor units and hence more muscle fibers. These cardiologists do not teach that the output of the organ of their speciality, the heart, determines the capacity of the skeletal muscles to produce force (as a result of a large cardiac output and hence a generous oxygen delivery to the exercising muscles). Rather they teach that the speed at which we run or the weight that we can lift, is determined by the number of motor units that are recruited in our exercising limbs. Exercise physiologists on the other hand consistently argue that how fast we run is determined solely by the magnitude of our maximal cardiac output [7, 8]. Most remain vigorously opposed to any suggestion that the extent of skeletal muscle recruitment plays any role.

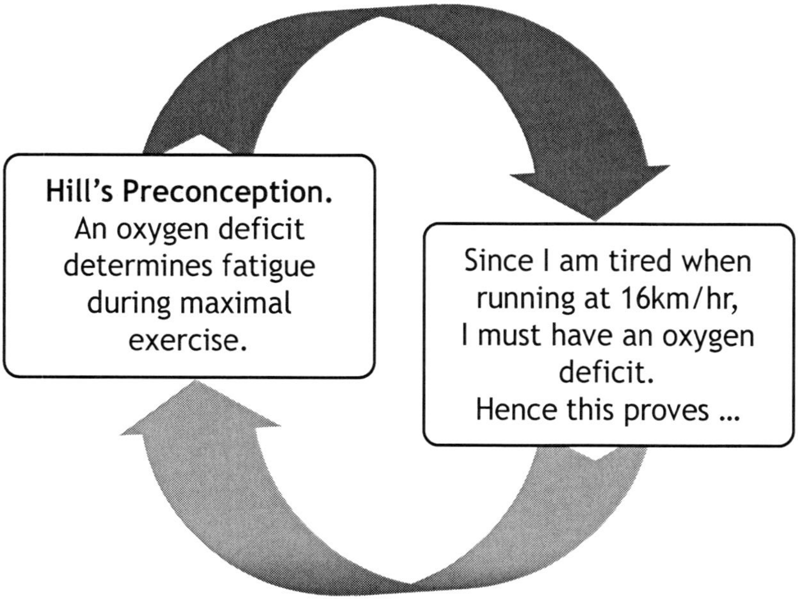

Figure 1. The circular logic on which A.V. Hill established his Cardiovascular/Anaerobic/Catastrophic Model of Human Exercise Performance.

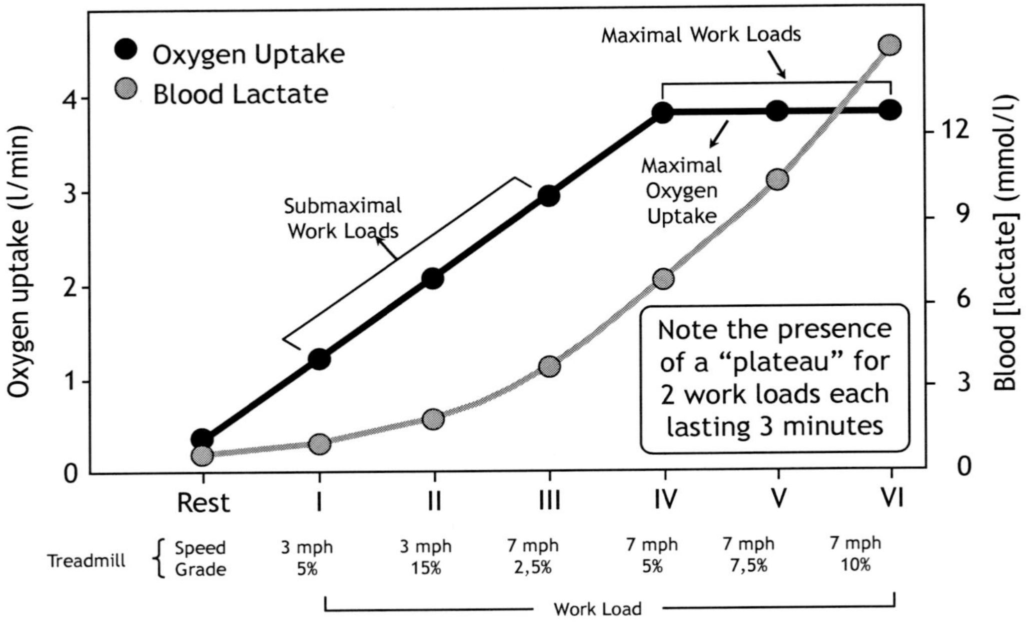

Figure 2. An early graphic depicting the "plateau phenomenon" according to the interpretation of Mitchell and Blomqvist in 1971.

After completing my Doctor of Medicine degree I began to teach courses in sports sciences and to establish a sports science laboratory. At the time it was believed that the measure of a proper exercise scientist was his or her proven ability accurately to measure the maximum oxygen consumption (VO_2max) of athletes. Furthermore, the more "elite" the athletes that he or she was able to test, the more important must be the exercise scientist. This perversity occurred because of the discipline-wide dogma that the VO_2max alone defines all there is to know about human exercise performance. Nothing else really mattered, then or even now [9].

Quite quickly I also learned that a study measuring the VO_2max could not be published in a reputable sports science journal at that time unless in included the following statement: "The plateau phenomenon was identified in 100% of tested subjects". However we were unable to identify this phenomenon in studies of rats [10, 11] and humans [12] with the regularity that the discipline then required. The challenge was either to follow this popular tendency and to write that which we had not found. Or else to discover why, uniquely in the entire world [8] it seems that we are the only researchers unable to discover this "plateau phenomenon" in 100% of our tested subjects.

Better to understand our unique failure, I became interested in the history of how this intimate linkage had developed between oxygen consumption, in particular the VO_2max, and athletic performance. One natural starting point was Professor David Costill's first book on the physiology of long distance running [13]. For at the time there was no exercise physiologist who better understood the application of exercise physiology to athletic performance. On page 26 I discovered the following statement: "Since the early work of Hill and Lupton [14], exercise physiologists have associated the limits of human endurance with the ability to consume larger volumes of oxygen during exhaustive exercise". This statement suggested that this linkage likely began with the work of the English physiologists Professor A.V. Hill and Dr Harry Lupton. My readings soon led me to a foundation study of Professor Frederick Gowland Hopkins of the University of Cambridge. This study was clearly pivotal in the evolution of Hill's beliefs.

By the time they reported their studies, Hill and Hopkins had both won Nobel prizes for Physiology or Medicine but neither was a neurophysiologist. Hopkins was a biochemist and Hill a muscle physiologist. It is perhaps natural that any models to understand human exercise performance that either developed would focus predominantly on biochemical and physiological explanations without any reference to the brain. Furthermore as Hill was essentially a muscle physiologist, since it was for the study of muscle that he had been awarded the Nobel Prize in 1922, it was to be expected that he would place skeletal muscle at the centre of any model of human exercise physiology that he developed.

The studies of Hopkins were particularly interesting because his intent was not to study exercise physiology in humans but rather to measure the true lactic acid concentrations in the skeletal muscles of recently dead creatures, specifically frogs. He had found that the lactate concentrations of frog skeletal muscle were never low under these conditions. He surmised that some chemical reaction was activated by death causing lactate concentrations to rise in muscles sampled after death. He soon discovered that muscle lactate concentrations were much lower when the harvested muscles were placed immediately in ice-cold alcohol, than they were in muscles not treated this way. Furthermore if the excised muscles were then stored in an atmosphere of nitrogen, their lactate concentrations continued to rise. Whereas, lactate concentrations fell progressively in muscles stored in oxygen. Hopkins and W.M. Fletcher, who is remembered as Hill's tutor, subsequently concluded that "lactic acid is spontaneously developed, under anaerobic conditions in excised muscle" and that "fatigue due to contractions is accompanied by an increase of lactic acid" [15].

In fact in the context of what he was studying, Hopkins should have concluded that "since lactic acid is spontaneously developed in excised frog muscle, so this reaction must be stopped by immediately placing the excised muscle in ice-cold alcohol if the true ante-mortem muscle lactate concentration is to be measured". Unfortunately this conclusion was not properly conveyed. As a consequence when A.V. Hill began to interpret his own findings, he quickly concluded that Hopkins' work had *proved* that skeletal muscles produce lactic acid *only* when they are "anaerobic" and that it is this production of lactic acid that *causes* skeletal muscle fatigue. The point of course is that Hopkins and Fletcher's work had essentially nothing to do with exercise physiology. They studied neither exercise, nor "anaerobiosis" (rather they studied totally anoxic muscle that did not have a blood supply). Nor did they even study mammals, let alone humans.

My readings led me ultimately to the critical statement by Hill, Long and Lupton [16] that: "Considering the case of running ... there is clearly some critical speed for each individual ... above which, the maximum oxygen intake is inadequate, lactic acid accumulating, a continuously increasing oxygen debt being incurred, fatigue and exhaustion setting in". Unrecognized at the time was that this interpretation introduced the novel concept of catastrophe into the teaching of physiology, more specifically into exercise physiology. For the standard teaching in human physiology is that the body has multiple redundant controls to ensure that all bodily systems are homeostatically regulated under all conditions of life [17] but fail catastrophically only at the moment of death. Yet in this single paragraph A.V. Hill introduced the concept of catastrophic failure into human exercise physiology. A measure of the resilience of his interpretation is that nearly 90 years later, this concept of fatigue resulting from a catastrophic physiological failure remains intact and largely unchallenged in almost all the teaching and writing in the exercise sciences.

At the 1987 American College of Sports Medicine Annual Conference I was invited to speak on the role of exercise testing for the prediction of athletic performance. There for the first time I showed that Hill's original study did not prove the conclusion that he had drawn (Figure 2 in [18]). Specifically that he had not established that fatigue during maximal exercise is caused by the development of anaerobiosis in the exercising muscles. By re-analyzing Hill's data, I was able to show that he had based his interpretation and hence built his entire cardiovascular/anaerobic/catastrophic (CAC) model on the basis of his preconceived belief that an oxygen deficit causes fatigue during maximal exercise (Figure 1). Yet the basis for his interpretation was the sensation of fatigue that he developed when running at the highest speeds of which he was capable. Thus when he experienced the symptoms of fatigue whilst running at 16 km/h, Hill assumed that he had suddenly developed an oxygen deficit. Hence the model that Hill conceived was entirely dependant on his preconception, even before he began his first experiment, that skeletal muscle anaerobiosis causes fatigue (Figure 1). As a result Hill's experiment simply "proved" what he already believed and did not consider any other possible explanations.

In 1971 J.H. Mitchell and G. Blomqvist [19] produced the classic figure, reproduced here as Figure 2, which indicated their interpretation of how the failure of oxygen delivery conceived by Hill, limits maximal exercise performance by producing a "plateau" in oxygen consumption. Notice that their depiction of a plateau was specific – the absence of any further increase in oxygen consumption once a maximum value had been achieved. Currently there are about 13 modern definitions of the criteria used to define the "plateau phenomenon" [1] and none describes the precise and unequivocal event depicted by Mitchell and Blomqvist in this figure. For if the "plateau phenomenon" is caused by the physiological phenomena that Hill described (and as detailed below), specifically the onset of myocardial ischaemia leading to skeletal muscle anaerobiosis, then the description of what constitutes a "plateau phenomenon" is quite simple – it must take the form depicted by Mitchell and Blomqvist.

But according to the Hill model the real test of a maximal effort must be the development of myocardial ischaemia, a point that is persistently avoided by those seeking to prove that a particular VO_2max measurement is truly "maximal" [20-24] (see also Chapter 5).

Hill's Understanding of the Factors Initiating and Terminating Skeletal Muscle Contraction

Hill's understanding of skeletal muscle contraction was the following: "When a muscle is stimulated, a certain amount of lactic acid is liberated at certain surfaces within it. This, by some physical or chemical process still uncertain, causes a development of force and, if allowed, a shortening of the muscle. The acid is then rapidly neutralized, its effect passes off, and the muscle relaxes. The process can be repeated again and again until the available supply of alkali for neutralizing the acid has been used up, when the rapidly increasing acidity of the muscle stops its further activity. This stage is that of complete fatigue, and the amount of work which the muscle can perform depends on the degree to which it can tolerate acid before this stage is reached".

"The acid slows the relaxation of the muscle. This last effect is very striking in short distance races. Where slower muscle relaxation, commencing within seven or eight seconds from the start, causes a progressive diminution in the maximum speed long before exhaustion. This formation of lactic acid is the chemical reaction on which the whole of voluntary muscular activity depends" [25] (p. 224-225).

Figure 3 shows the mechanism of fatigue according to Hill's model of exercise physiology as I understood it up to 1996 and as is usually taught in the majority of modern textbooks of exercise physiology. The key concept is that there is a maximum or limiting cardiac output which cannot be exceeded. As a result there is a limit to the amount of blood that can be pumped to the exercising muscles. But during maximal exercise, the exercising muscles' requirement for blood flow exceed this maximal rate. As a result the muscle begins to function "anaerobically" with the production of lactic acid in excess. This lactic acid inhibits muscle contraction, in fact muscle relaxation according to Hill's original understanding.

That this is still the accepted explanation is shown by the statement in the most current review of "what do we know and what do we still need to know" about the VO_2max: "the primary distinguishing characteristic of elite endurance athletes that allows them to run fast over prolonged periods of time is a large, compliant heart with a compliant pericardium that can accommodate a lot of blood, very fast, to take advantage of the Starling mechanism to generate a large stroke volume" [7] (p. 31).

But my conclusion in a presentation at the 1987 ACSM conference was that: "Yet a critical review of Hill and Lupton's results shows that they inferred but certainly did not prove that oxygen limitations develop during maximal exercise... This review proposes that the factors limiting maximal exercise performance might be better explained in terms of a failure of muscle contractility ("muscle power"), which may be independent of tissue oxygen deficiency. The implications for exercise testing and the prediction of athletic performance are discussed" [18].

My reference to the potential role of changes in muscle contractility in regulating maximal exercise performance was based on (i) my training in cardiac physiology and (ii) my assumption, shared with all exercise scientists at that time (and still assumed by all those who like Levine [7] and Shephard [8] believed in a peripheral regulation of exercise performance), that fatigue in any form of exercise, regardless of duration or intensity, must occur only *after* all the available motor units in the exercising limbs have been recruited. It was natural to draw this conclusion since this was the presumption that all exercise physiologists shared at that time. For the simple reason that if exercise is regulated purely by changes in the ability of the exercising skeletal muscles to produce force, so called peripheral fatigue, then fatigue can only occur once all the available motor units have been activated in the exercising limbs. For if this is not the case and if exercise terminates *before* all the motor units and hence muscle fibers have been activated in the exercising limbs, then the brain must be the regulator of the exercise performance. For it has caused the exercise to terminate prematurely (by mechanisms still unknown) even when fresh, non-fatigued muscle fibers remain in the exercising limbs. This peripheral fatigue/regulation model cannot explain how exercise can terminate even though there is a population of fresh, unused skeletal muscle fibers in the exercising limbs waiting to be recruited.

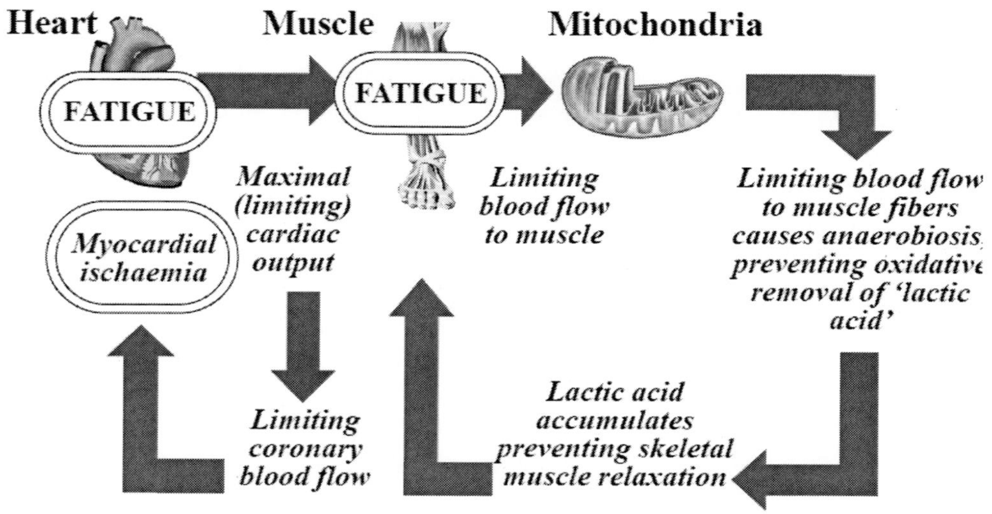

Figure 3. The sequence of physiological events that are usually considered to cause fatigue during progressive maximal exercise to exhaustion according to the popular interpretation of the A.V. Hill model.

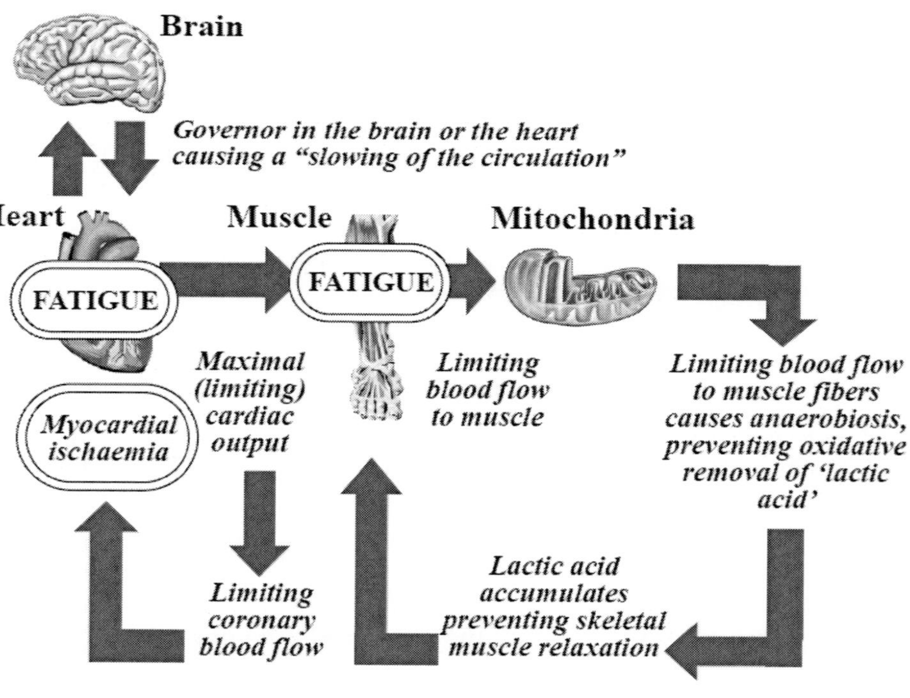

Figure 4. The real sequence of physiological events that A.V. Hill and colleagues described in 1923 as the cause of fatigue during progressive maximal exercise to exhaustion.

Nine years later in the 1996 J.B. Wolffe Memorial Lecture I proposed "...an alternate physiological model ... in which skeletal muscle contractile activity is regulated by a series of central, predominantly neural, and peripheral, predominantly chemical, regulators that act to prevent the development of organ damage or even death during exercise in both health and disease and under demanding environmental conditions....Regulation of skeletal muscle contractile function by central mechanisms would prevent the development of hypotension and myocardial ischemia during exercise in persons with heart failure, of hyperthermia during exercise in the heat, and of cerebral hypoxia during exercise at extreme altitude" [26]. Once again my theory was based on my continuing assumption that fatigue during any form of exercise must occur only after there is complete (total) skeletal muscle recruitment in the exercising limbs.

This paper was rebutted by Drs. David Bassett and Edward Howley of the University of Tennessee who concluded that: "When we weigh the scientific evidence on both sides of the issue, it appears that Hill's views were amazingly accurate. Scientific investigations in the 70 years since Hill have served mainly to reinforce his paradigms and confirm that his scientific "hunches" were correct. Only relatively minor refinements to his theories have been needed. In contrast Noakes' views are not supported by strong scientific evidence, and they raised numerous paradoxes and unresolved dilemmas" [27].

This rebuttal encouraged me once again to review all of Hill's writings. I discovered a critical paragraph that had been overlooked by all previous authors including myself: "The enormous output of the hearts of an able-bodied men, maintained for considerable periods during vigorous exercise, requires a large contemporary supply of oxygen to meet the demands for energy... . When the oxygen supply becomes inadequate, it is probable that the heart rapidly begins to diminish its output, so avoiding exhaustion" [16]. Hill next suggested a mechanism which would prevent the development of irreversible heart damage during maximal exercise: "We suggest that ... either in the heart muscle itself or in the nervous system, there is some mechanism (a governor) which causes a slowing of the circulation as soon as a serious degree of unsaturation occurs". Remarkably Hill foresaw that this mechanism acted in an anticipatory manner even though it was activated only after the catastrophe had already begun. The function of this anticipatory control was to insure that a worse catastrophe, irreversible myocardial damage, was prevented.

Unfortunately Hill did not indicate in which organ system or at which site he believed this "serious degree of unsaturation" was detected, activating this anticipatory reflex. Was the oxygenation of the skeletal muscles or the heart or perhaps even the brain threatened? A "dangerous degree of unsaturation" cannot occur in the systemic *arterial* circulation including the circulation to the coronary arteries supplying the heart muscle, or to the skeletal muscles or perhaps even to the brain unless the exercise is performed at extreme altitude or if there is co-existing lung disease, both of which cause the arterial oxygen partial pressure to fall especially during exercise. Hill seems not have understood this. Probably he conceived that maximal exercise caused oxygen "unsaturation" in the active tissues and that this "unsaturation" adversely affected the function, first of the heart and then as a consequence, of the skeletal muscles. Ninety years later we cannot be sure of exactly what Hill believed [28].

But we do now know that myocardial "unsaturation" (ischaemia) must occur if the cardiac output reaches a truly maximal value whilst the exercise intensity continues to increase. This is because myocardial perfusion is critically dependant on the coronary perfusion pressure [29] which cannot increase once a truly maximal cardiac output has been reached. Instead coronary perfusion must fall leading to a progressive myocardial ischaemia. My interpretation of what I believe Hill meant is shown in Figure 4. In this model the heart and brain are in communication in order to produce a reduction in myocardial function as soon as the myocardial ischaemia that Hill predicted must develop, happens. Again a critical consequence of this model was to introduce the concept of catastrophic failure into human exercise physiology.

The moment I understood Hill's model, my training in cardiovascular physiology made me realize that the human body would not have survived the selective pressures of evolution if it had been designed in this way. Instead of the brain protecting the heart by reducing myocardial function directly, as Hill described, the more effective method of control would be to reduce the demands placed on the heart by the action of the exercising muscles. Thus Figure 5 shows the essential modifications to Hill's original "governor" theory that converted it into the CGM. By regulating the amount of muscle recruited by the brain in a feed forward manner on a moment-to-moment basis, the central nervous system can insure that homeostasis is maintained in all bodily systems, not just the heart.

Figure 6 shows that sections of the original A.V. Hill model are usually studied by scientists working in different sub-disciplines in the exercise sciences. These sub-disciplines include muscle physiology, biochemistry, applied sports science, cardiovascular and respiratory physiology, neurophysiology and in some cases even statistics [30]. The problem is that protagonists of each of these sub-disciplines tend to see only that part of the model that falls within their ambit of expertise and understanding.

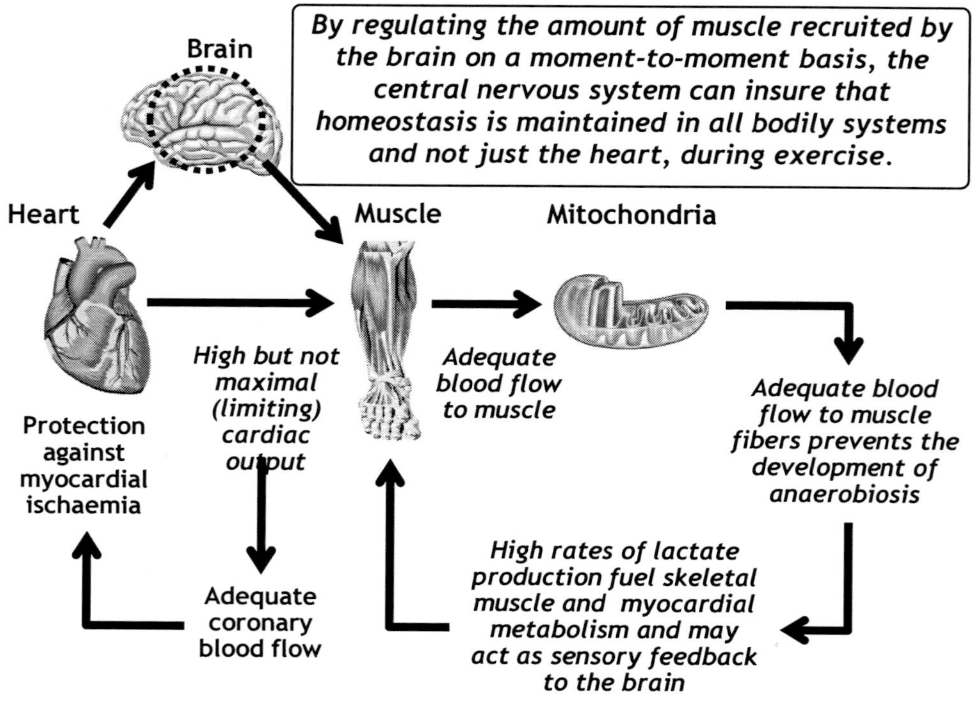

Figure 5. The modified model – the Central Governor Model – that evolved from A.V. Hill's model (Figure 4).

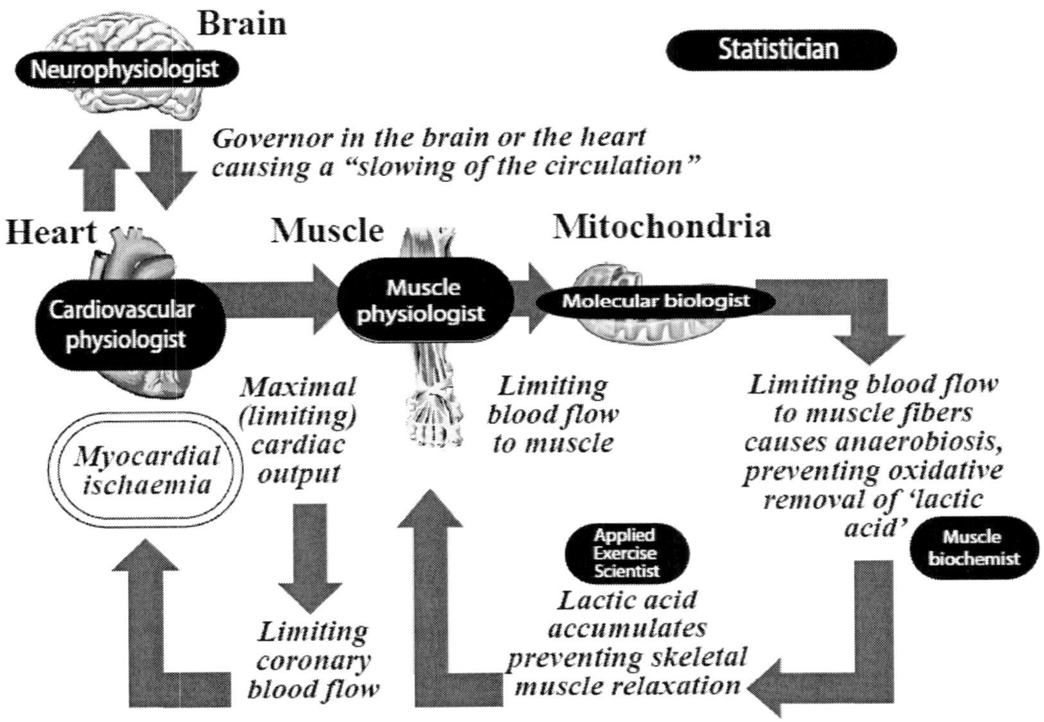

Figure 6. Exercise scientists tend to explain fatigue and exercise performance on the basis of the functioning of the organ systems, tissues or molecular mechanisms that fall within their specific areas of expertise.

Thus, for example, scientists trained in cardiovascular physiology are more likely to develop a model of exercise physiology in which the heart and cardiovascular system are the dominant players [7, 8, 19, 21, 22, 31, 32]. As a result they tend to assume that an understanding of human exercise performance can be acquired purely by understanding the cardiovascular response to exercise. In contrast biochemists will usually argue that fatigue can be described purely on the basis of known biochemical changes in the body during exercise whereas muscle physiologists and applied exercise scientists will imagine that all fatigue must originate in skeletal muscle [20, 27, 33-36]. For the truth is what we study and what we believe, is determined by our area of interest (and expertise). And often what we believe is determined by what we believed even before we began our research.

But the problem is that the body does not function in discrete, disconnected compartments and so cannot be studied as if it does by scientists with a compartmentalized understanding of human physiology. Nor will such compartmentalized study force the body to act that way, however much we might wish it.

Undoubtedly the most damaging effect of the A.V. Hill model, other than the development of the concept of fatigue as a form of catastrophe failure, has been to exclude central command from the brain as a possible factor determining exercise performance [37]. Thus his specific physiological model of fatigue focused the minds of generations of exercise scientists on maximal exercise to exhaustion in the laboratory as the dominant (and simplest) model for the study of fatigue. Yet in this model the experimenter controls the athlete's level of central command by progressively increasing the work rate. As a result the only manner in which the tested subject's brain can influence the exercise performance is either by increasing the extent of skeletal muscle recruitment in the active limbs (in response to the externally-driven, progressive increase in the work rate) or by terminating the exercise. There are no other options. Thus since it is the controlled variable in the experiment, the role of central command in regulating the exercise performance cannot be determined by this testing method. Only when the athlete is allowed to set her own pace does the role of central command in the regulation of the exercise behavior become obvious [38, 39].

TWO COMPETING MODELS TO EXPLAIN EITHER THE LIMITATION (A.V. HILL MODEL) OR THE REGULATION (CENTRAL GOVERNOR MODEL) OF HUMAN EXERCISE PERFORMANCE

Figure 7 shows the main features of the two competing models that are currently used to explain the factors that either limit or regulate human exercise performance. The A.V.Hill CAC or homeostatic failure model is based on the use of a series of fixed but increasing work rates set by the experimenter, and which continue to increase until the tested subject is no longer able further to increase the work rate at which point the exercise test terminates.

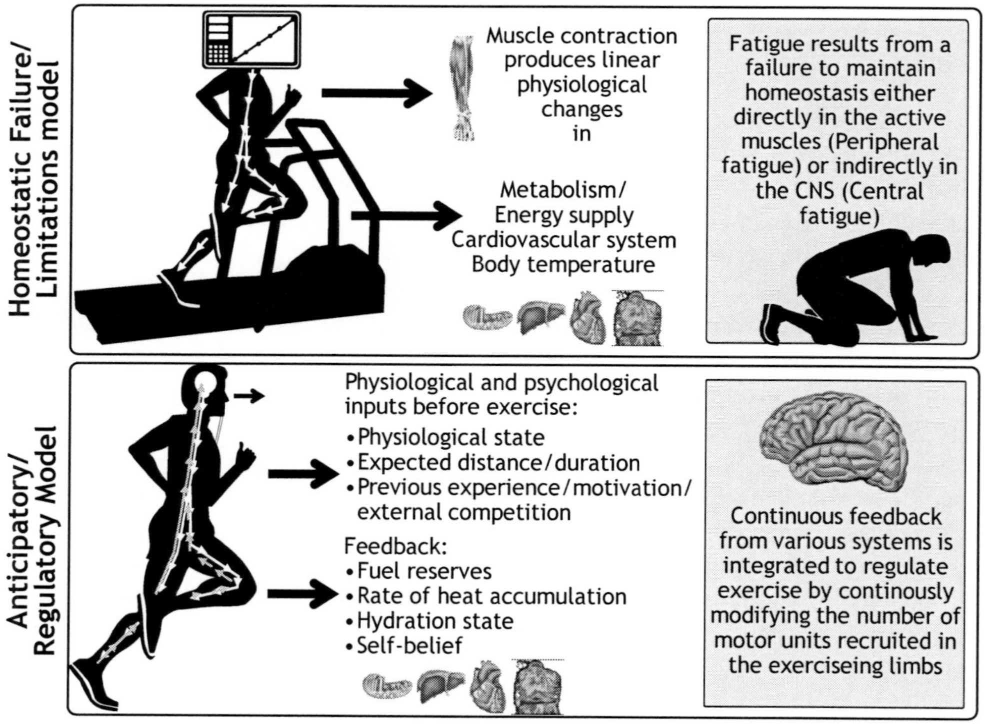

Figure 7. Two opposing models – the homeostatic failure/limitations model or the anticipatory regulatory model (CGM) - are currently used to explain human exercise performance.

The interpretation then is that muscle contraction produces linear physiological changes in metabolism, in energy provision, and in the cardiovascular, respiratory, thermoregulatory and hormonal responses, amongst many others. Ultimately one or more systems fail as each is unable further to increase its functional capacity in response to another increase in the work rate. Rather the exercise must terminate as soon as the maximal functional capacity of one or more systems has been exceeded. As a result, fatigue is caused by a failure to maintain homeostasis either directly in the active muscles (peripheral fatigue) or indirectly in the central nervous system (central fatigue). Note that this model does not include any role for feedback from the periphery to influence the extent of central motor command. My contention is that an unquestioning devotion to this form of testing has produced the "brainless" model of exercise physiology that we currently teach since in this form of testing the usual function of the tested subject's brain to establish the pacing strategy is usurped by the brain of the experimenter [37]. Thus the role of the brain in determining the exercise performance cannot be detected during the VO_2max test.

In contrast the anticipatory model allows feedback from the periphery to influence the extent of the feed forward central command that determines the level of skeletal muscle recruitment. Thus this model allows the action of physiological and psychological inputs before exercise to establish the athlete's initial pace. These factors likely include the athlete's physiological state at the start of exercise; the expected distance or duration of the intended exercise bout; the degree of previous experience that the athlete has, most especially in the specific activity that is being undertaken; the athlete's level of motivation which will be critically influenced by the level of external competition and the importance the athlete ascribes to the event; as well as the athlete's level of self-belief amongst many other psychological factors.

Then during the exercise, there will be continuous feedback from all the organs in the body which will inform the central command of the state of the fuel reserves, the rate of heat accumulation and the hydration state, amongst a host of many other factors.

Table 1. How do the A.V. Hill and Central Governor Models explain some common phenomena observed in athletes?

Phenomenon	**Peripheral Model**	**Central Governor Model**
Pacing	One pace for all distances	Variable pacing
End spurt	Impossible	Possible
Homeostasis	Fatigue due to loss of homeostasis	Homeostasis maintained under all conditions as a result of behavior modification
Skeletal muscle activation	Exercise terminates with 100% muscle activation	Never 100% muscle activation during exercise
Drug effects	Act on heart, lungs, muscles, but not brain	Explains effects of drugs acting on brain
RPE	A measure of the exercise intensity	A measure of the relative exercise duration

As a result continuous feedback from all these systems is integrated to regulate exercise by continuously modifying the number of motor units recruited in the exercising limbs. That this system allows an anticipatory regulation of the exercise performance is the central prediction of the CGM and which distinguishes it from the traditional central fatigue model [40, 41] which acknowledges that the brain is responsible for the termination of exercise but only after there has been some catastrophic failure of brain function. In other words, the central fatigue model as originally conceived lacked any reference to the brain's ability to anticipate a future failure and to insure that the exercise behaviour was modified specifically to insure that homeostasis was protected and a catastrophic failure prevented.

The Explanation for Six Common Exercise Phenomena according to either the Limitation (A. V. Hill Model) or the Regulation (Central Governor Model (CGM)) of Human Exercise Performance

Table 1 lists six phenomena that must be obvious to all who study human exercise physiology [42]. It includes the explanation for these phenomena according to either the A.V. Hill or the Central Governor Model (CGM). With regard to the first phenomenon, pacing, only the CGM can explain the variable pacing strategy that is observed in all sporting competitions [43, 44] and indeed in the moment to moment changes in muscle power output during exercise [45]. In contrast the Hill model predicts that athletes can only ever follow one pacing strategy. Specifically one in which they begin exercise at an unsustainable pace that then slows as the negative pacing molecule, lactate, begins to accumulate causing the progressive slowing as described by Hill in 1923.

There is growing interest in the concept that Homo sapiens evolved from Homo habilis as a result of the persistence hunting to their exhaustion (as a result of hyperthermic paralysis) of large, faster moving antelope in conditions of extreme heat [46-48]. Thus the current theory is that between 2 to 3 million years ago early hominids learned how to hunt animals to their extinction by chasing each until its body temperature was abnormally elevated causing paralysis. When paralyzed, the antelope could be dispatched without the use of metal-tipped spears which were first constructed only about 60,000 years ago. As a result according to this theory for 2 million years or more, early hominids were able to kill with their bare hands large antelope protected by dangerous horns. The high protein diets provided by the capture of this energy rich food would explain the increase in brain size that occurred especially over the last 500,000 years.

In order to capture the antelope under these conditions, human persistence hunters would have had to evolve a complex anticipatory pacing strategy in which they retained sufficient reserves not just for the 4-6 hours that they chased those antelope but also for the period that would be required to carry the captured meat back to their hungry families.

One of the clearest studies showing the presence of this anticipatory pacing was reported by Amann et al [49] although the authors perhaps undervalued the physiological relevance of their finding [50]. Figure 8 shows that their study found evidence for anticipatory pacing beginning within less than 60 seconds of exposure, without their knowledge, to gas mixtures with different inspired oxygen fractions (FiO_2). The effect was dose-dependent and was greatest when subjects were exposed to an FiO_2 of 15%. Importantly EMG activity during exercise at different FiO_2 was reduced in proportion to the reductions in power output indicating that (i) that the reduction in power output on exposure to hypoxia was associated, as predicted by the CGM, with a reduced central command and (ii) this effect was anticipatory and did not occur only after there had already been some catastrophic failure (as a result of the development of severe hypoxia in one or more critical organs). Furthermore under all conditions there was the presence of an "end spurt" in which the subjects increased their power outputs. The endspurt occurred also with an increase in EMG activity in the active skeletal muscles, indicating that the endspurt was also due to an increased central command (as predicted by the CGM). Indeed the second and perhaps one of the most interesting phenomena in exercise physiology is this "end spurt" in which athletes like Haile Gebrselassie (Figure 9) speed up at the end of the race, running the fastest when they should be the most tired [43].

The end spurt phenomenon poses significant theoretical problems for our current understanding of fatigue which is most simply defined as an inability to maintain the present or required work rate. Yet elite athletes like Gebrselassie cannot be fatigued according to this definition if they are able to speed up at the end of their world record-setting performances. Thus this simple observation poses a real problem for our current understanding of fatigue. It cannot continue to be ignored simply because it is inconvenient.

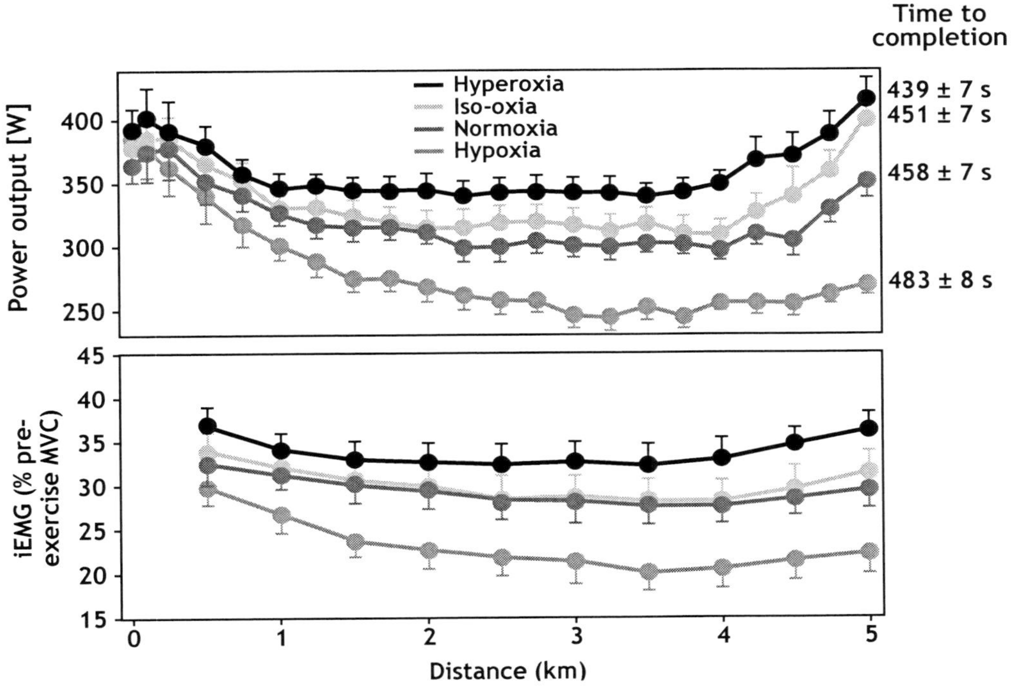

Figure 8. Effect of different inspired oxygen fractions on power output (top panel) and muscle activation (integrated EMG (iEMG) activity as a % of that achieved during an MVC) during 5km cycling time trials. The study shows the presence of anticipatory pacing strategies present within the first km of the trial and the end spurt beginning after 4km..

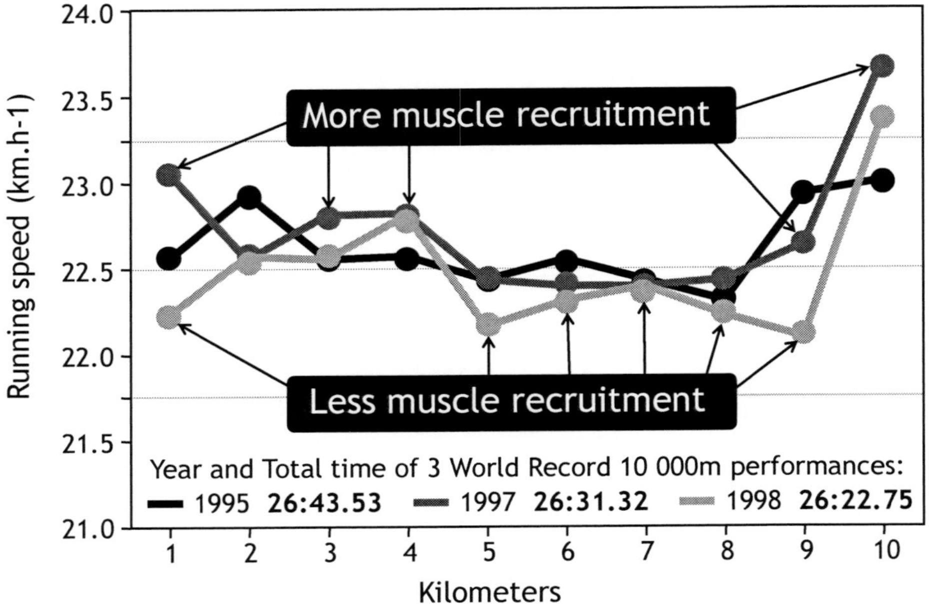

Figure 9. Running speeds for each kilometer during 3 world 10 000m record performances by Ethiopia's Haille Gebrsellasie. Note the presence of a marked end spurt in each race. According to the CGM, the different paces are due to continual, moment-to-moment changes in the levels of skeletal muscle recruitment with reduced recruitment in the middle of the race and increased recruitment in the endspurt during the final 1 km.

According to the CGM, the moment to moment [45] changes in pacing strategies that occur during exercise are due to changes in the extent of skeletal muscle recruitment (Figure 9), either increased or decreased according to whether the athlete speeds up or slows down. Thus according to the CGM, the end spurt is due to the recruitment of additional skeletal muscle motor units in the exercising limbs as the end of exercise approaches. The point of course is that the Hill CAC model cannot explain the end spurt phenomenon any more effectively than it can explain how the pacing strategy is set at the start of exercise [42].

The third phenomenon is the protection of homoeostasis which, according to the Hill model, does not occur. Rather according to that model it is the failure of homeostasis that causes fatigue and exhaustion. In contrast the key prediction of the CGM is that behaviour modification insures that homoeostasis is protected under all conditions. Thus the CGM treats exercise as a behaviour that is continuously modified to insure that cellular homoeostasis is protected under all conditions. Indeed many presentations at this conference will evaluate behavior modifications the goal of which appear to be the maintenance of homeostasis during exercise.

The fourth phenomenon is the difference in the extent of skeletal muscle activation that the either model predict is present at the point of fatigue. As already argued, the Hill model predicts that exercise must terminate when there is 100% activation of all the motor units in the exercising limbs. For the simple reason that if the periphery alone determines the exercise performance, then the activity must continue until all the muscle fibers have been recruited and exercised to the point of their individual exhaustion. Whereas the CGM predicts that

100% muscle activation does not occur in any form of exercise since this is likely to threaten homeostasis and cause bodily damage.

There is convincing evidence that skeletal muscle recruitment is never 100% except perhaps in medical conditions such as infection with the tetanus bacillus which causes tetanic muscle contractions that may lead to bony fractures [51-53]. Similarly treatment of schizophrenia with the analeptic (convulsion-producing) drug, metrazol [54, 55], or of depression with convulsive shock therapy [56] was associated with bony fractures before these forms of treatment were finally terminated. The point of these examples is that if unregulated skeletal muscle contraction can produce sufficient force to cause bony fractures, then it makes sense that complete skeletal muscle recruitment must be prevented by some central control mechanism.

The fifth phenomenon is the manner in which certain drugs that act only on the central nervous system can improve exercise performance. According to the Hill model drugs that improve exercise performance must act on the heart, lungs and the muscles but not on the brain since, according to the "brainless" model of human exercise performance (Figure 2 in Chapter 5), the brain plays no part in such performance. In contrast the CGM is able to explain why certain drugs that act exclusively on the brain can improve exercise performance. Our own studies show that amphetamines act by reducing the extent of skeletal muscle reserve and therefore allow exercise to continue for longer at a higher intensity [57].

When I began to write more widely on the CGM I received the following personal correspondence from a former professional cyclist. He wrote: "If I go and inject myself with 250 mg of speed amphetamines the drug will have a rapid effect on this governor and I can guarantee that I will have God-like strength that was there all along but I was never able to access before as my governor is a tight bastard! The only limiter will be when I drop dead or run out of fuel. Unfortunately for me I've seen both sides of the effects of drugs in sport. My wife's previous boyfriend died from racing in hot conditions whilst under the influence (of amphetamines). Super natural rides used to be common here until drug testing came and they all had to switch to more subtle expensive products".

The sixth phenomenon is the rating of perceived exertion (RPE) which according to the classic interpretation of its originator, Dr Gunnar Borg, is a measure exclusively of the exercise intensity [58]. In contrast in developing the CGM, we discovered that the RPE is a measure of the duration of exercise that has been completed or that which remains [59]. I first became aware of this possibility when I evaluate the study of Baldwin and colleagues [60] and found that their data showed a significant linear relationship between the RPE and the exercise duration [61]. Furthermore the rate at which the RPE rose was greater when the subjects were carbohydrate-depleted than when they began exercise with intact carbohydrate stores. But when the RPE data were plotted against the relative, rather than the absolute exercise duration, all the data points fell on the same line indicating the presence of a fundamental biological law: Specifically that the RPE rises as a function of the expected exercise duration.

We have since shown that the RPE is different from the start of exercise in the heat even though the rectal temperatures were not different at that time [62]. Therefore the brain had calculated the projected rate of heat retention in different environmental conditions and had planned, in anticipation, the exercise duration that could be safely sustained without the risk that heat stroke would develop.

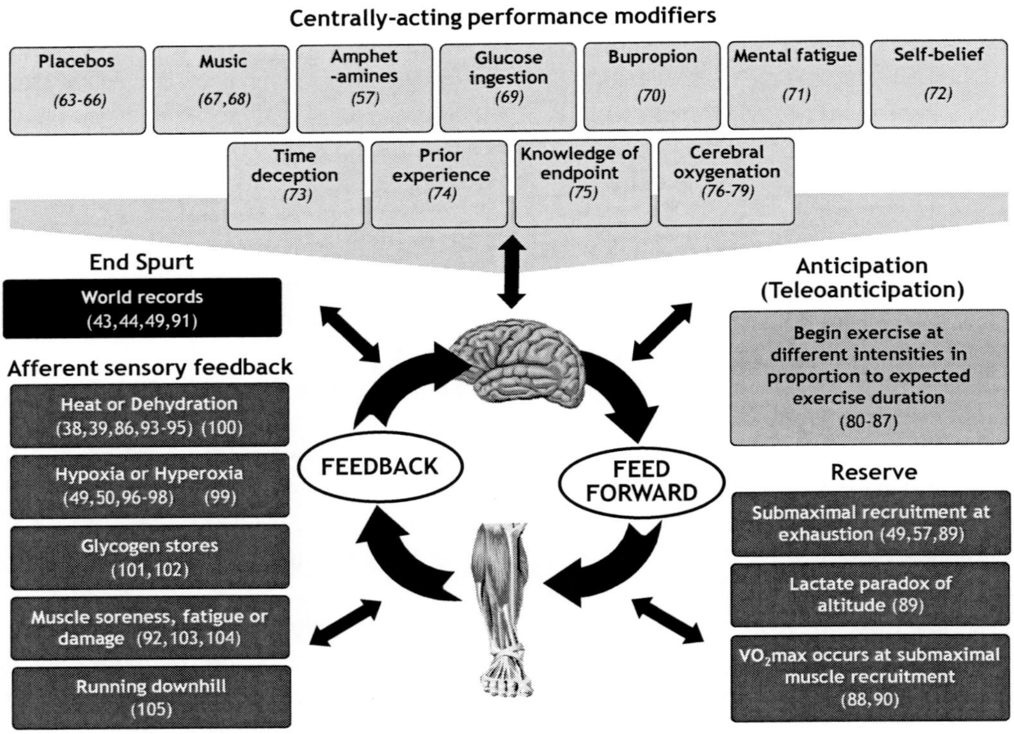

Figure 10. Recent studies that are compatible with the functioning of a CGM but which cannot be explained by the A.V. Hill model. The numbers refer to the reference number for each cited study.

In summary, there are 6 phenomena, well-known to all who observe or study exercise, that cannot be adequately explained by the traditional Hill CAC model but which are compatible with the predictions of the CGM. When added to the compelling body of evidence that disproves the biological basis for the Hill model [1], it becomes quite difficult to understand how some [8] continue to argue with great vehemence, that it is the CGM not the Hill model that needs to be "retired".

Some Current Studies which Confirm that Exercise is Regulated in Anticipation by Central Motor Command that Responds also to the Presence of Feedback from a Variety of Peripheral Organs

Figure 10 shows some of the key predictions of the CGM. These are (i) that the ultimate regulation of the exercise performance resides in the central nervous system, the function of which is potentially modifiable by interventions that act exclusively on central (brain) mechanisms; (ii) that the exercise pace is set "in anticipation"; (iii) that the protection of homeostasis requires that there is always a skeletal muscle reserve during all forms of exercise; (iv) that the exercise intensity may increase near the end of exercise – the end spurt even in the face of significant "fatigue"; and (v) that afferent sensory feedback can modify the exercise performance.

Thus in the very recent past a series of studies have shown that exercise performance can be modified by a number of interventions that act solely on the central nervous system including placebos [63-66], music [67, 68], the amphetamines [57], glucose ingestion [69], bupropion [70], mental fatigue [71], self-belief [72], time deception [73], prior experience [74], knowledge of the endpoint of exercise [75] and altered cerebral oxygenation reduced by beta-adrenergic blockade [76], heat [77], maximal exercise [78] and hypoxic exercise [79]. Similarly the evidence for the anticipatory control of exercise [80-87], for skeletal muscle reserve during exercise [57, 88-90], the end spurt [43, 44, 49, 91], and for afferent sensory feedback related to prior exercise [92], to exercise in the heat [38, 39, 86, 93-95], in hypoxia [49, 50, 96-98] or alternatively hyperoxia [99], the extent of dehydration [100] and the body glycogen reserves [101, 102], muscle soreness [103] and muscle damage [104] or alternatively the act of running downhill [105], continues to accumulate.

Thus it would seem that the evidence to support a central control of exercise is rather more secure than is the (absence of firm evidence) on which Hill's CAC model is based [1].

Conclusion

The CGM views exercise as a behaviour that is regulated in anticipation by complex intelligent systems, the function of which are to ensure that whole body homoeostasis is protected under all conditions. This complexity cannot be appreciated if the body is studied as a collection of disconnected components as has become the usual practice in the modern exercise sciences.

Indeed on the basis of their work with US military conscripts during the Second World War, Bean and Eichna [106] warned already in 1943 that: "... physical fitness cannot be defined nor can differences be detected by means of a few simple physiological measurements ... obtained during limited tests ... . To do so results in focusing attention on some erroneous concept. Man is not a pulse rate, a rectal temperature, but a complex array of many phenomena.... Into performance enters the baffling yet extremely important factor of motivation, the will-to-do. This cannot be measured and remains an uncontrollable, quickly fluctuating, disturbing variable which may at any time completely alter the performance regardless of physical or physiologic state."

Similarly the medical student who was the first to break the four minute mile, Roger Bannister wrote in 1956 [107] that: "The human body is centuries in advance of the physiologist, and can perform an integration of heart, lungs and muscles which is too complex for the scientist to analyse". Later he continued: "It is the brain not the heart or lungs, that is the critical organ, it's the brain" [108]. Future generations of exercise scientists would be well advised to head the words of these most observant scientists.

The novel concepts predicted by the CGM [109, 110] and which are the opposite of those flowing from Hill's CAC model are the following:

1. The physiology of pacing, not fatigue, is the core issue for understanding exercise performance. The goal of pacing is to maintain homoeostasis and to prevent a catastrophic physiological failure.
2. Multiple, independent systems in the periphery provide sensory information that influences central motor command in the brain. The sum of this information generated in the center and in the periphery determines the pacing strategy during exercise.
3. Fatigue is purely a sensory perception which may be expressed physically as an alteration in the pacing strategy. Fatigue may therefore be a measure of the central neural efforts to maintain homoeostasis.
4. The role of the brain is to ensure that exhaustion develops and exercise terminates even though homoeostasis is maintained. As a result, a catastrophic outcome is prevented. This interpretation conflict absolutely with the traditional Hill model which predicts that exercise terminates only after there has been a failure of homeostasis in some bodily system.

The importance of this conference is that it will allow rigorous, open debate of an idea that challenges the very core of what is currently taught in the exercise sciences.

Like all theories that challenge an existing and entrenched dogma, the CGM has evoked a wave of distrust and many active attempts at its suppression. But the task of real science is to discover that which is true and so to advance our knowledge, not to attempt to suppress that which is inconvenient.

In his triology devoted to the study of the scientific process and those who produce new knowlege, Daniel J. Boorstein wrote that: “The barrier to knowledge is not ignorance. It is the illusion of knowledge”.

It is improbable that on the basis of the few simple experiments that he conducted, Professor Hill could have developed a model of exercise for which in the past 90 years “only relatively minor refinements to his theories have been needed” [9].

REFERENCES

[1] Noakes TD, St Clair Gibson A. Logical limitations to the "catastrophe" models of fatigue during exercise in humans. *Br J Sports Med*, 2004, 38, 648-9.

[2] Cooper D. *Chris Barnard by those who know him*. Vlaeberg, Cape Town, S.A.: Vlaeberg Publishers; 1992.

[3] Noakes TD, Opie LH. Substrates for maximum mechanical function in isolated perfused working rat heart. *J Appl Card*, 1989, 4, 391-405.

[4] Resink TJ, Gevers W, Noakes TD. Effects of extracellular calcium concentrations on myosin P light chain phosphorylation in hearts from running-trained rats. *J Mol Cell Cardiol*, 1981, 13, 753-65.

[5] Resink TJ, Gevers W, Noakes TD, Opie LH. Increased cardiac myosin ATPase activity as a biochemical adaptation to running training: enhanced response to catecholamines and a role for myosin phosphorylation. *J Mol Cell Cardiol*, 1981, 13, 679-94.

[6] Katz AM. *Physiology of the heart*. New York: Raven Press; 1977.

[7] Levine BD. VO2max: What do we know, and what do we still need to know? *J Physiol*, 2008, 586, 25-34.
[8] Shephard RJ. Is it time to retire the 'central governor'? *Sports Med*, 2009, 39, 709-21.
[9] McLaughlin JE, Howley ET, Bassett DR, Jr., Thompson DL, Fitzhugh EC. Test of the classic model for predicting endurance running performance. *Med Sci Sports Exerc*, 2010, 42, 991-7.
[10] Lambert MI, Noakes TD. Spontaneous running increases VO2max and running performance in rats. *J Appl Physiol*, 1990, 68, 400-3.
[11] Lambert MI, Noakes TD. Dissociation of changes in VO2 max, muscle QO2, and performance with training in rats. *J Appl Physiol*, 1989, 66, 1620-5.
[12] Noakes TD, Myburgh KH, Schall R. Peak treadmill running velocity during the VO2 max test predicts running performance. *J Sports Sci*, 1990, 8, 35-45.
[13] Costill DL. *A scientific approach to distance running*. Los Altos, California: Track and Field News; 1979.
[14] Hill AV, Lupton H. Muscular exercise, lactic acid, and the supply and utilization of oxygen. *Quart J Med*, 1923, 16, 135-71.
[15] Fletcher WM, Hopkins WG. Lactic acid in amphibian muscle. *J Physiol*, 1907, 35, 247-309.
[16] Hill AV, Long CHN, Lupton H. Muscular exercise, lactic acid and the supply and utilisation of oxygen: parts VII-VIII. *Proc Royal Soc Bri*, 1924, 97, 155-76.
[17] Lambert EV, St Clair GA, Noakes TD. Complex systems model of fatigue: integrative homoeostatic control of peripheral physiological systems during exercise in humans. *Br J Sports Med*, 2005, 39, 52-62.
[18] Noakes TD. Implications of exercise testing for prediction of athletic performance: a contemporary perspective. *Med Sci Sports Exerc*, 1988, 20, 319-30.
[19] Mitchell JH, Blomqvist G. Maximal oxygen uptake. *New Engl J Med*, 1971, 284, 1018-22.
[20] Hawkins MN, Snell PG, Stray-Gundersen J, Levine BD, Raven PB. Maximal oxygen uptake as a parametric measure of cardiorespiratory capacity. *Med Sci Sports Exerc*, 2007, 39, 103-7.
[21] Brink-Elfegoun T, Kaijser L, Gustafsson T, Ekblom B. Maximal oxygen uptake is not limited by a central nervous system governor. *J Appl Physiol*, 2007, 102, 781-6.
[22] Brink-Elfegoun T, Holmberg HC, Ekblom MN, Ekblom B. Neuromuscular and circulatory adaptation during combined arm and leg exercise with different maximal work loads. *Eur J Appl Physiol*, 2007, 101, 603-11.
[23] Day JR, Rossiter HB, Coats EM, Skasick A, Whipp BJ. The maximally attainable VO2 during exercise in humans: the peak vs. maximum issue. *J Appl Physiol*, 2003, 95, 1901-7.
[24] Rossiter HB, Kowalchuk JM, Whipp BJ. A test to establish maximum O2 uptake despite no plateau in the O2 uptake response to ramp incremental exercise. *J Appl Physiol*, 2006, 100, 764-70.
[25] Hill AV. The scientific study of athletics. *Sci Am*, 1926, 224-5.
[26] Noakes TD. Challenging beliefs: ex Africa semper aliquid novi: 1996 J.B. Wolffe Memorial Lecture. *Med Sci Sports Exerc*, 1997, 29, 571-90.
[27] Bassett DR, Jr., Howley ET. Maximal oxygen uptake: "classical" versus "contemporary" viewpoints. *Med Sci Sports Exerc*, 1997, 29, 591-603.

[28] Noakes TD. How did A V Hill understand the VO2max and the "plateau phenomenon"? Still no clarity? *Br J Sports Med*, 2008, 42, 574-80.
[29] Duncker DJ, Bache RJ. Regulation of coronary blood flow during exercise. *Physiol Rev*, 2008, 88, 1009-86.
[30] Hopkins WG. The improbable central governor of maximal endurance performance. *Sportscience*, 2009, 13, 9-12.
[31] Gonzalez-Alonso J, Calbet JA. Reductions in systemic and skeletal muscle blood flow and oxygen delivery limit maximal aerobic capacity in humans. *Circulation*, 2003, 107, 824-30.
[32] Mitchell JH, Saltin B. The oxygen transport system and maximal oxygen uptake. In: Tipton CM, editor. *Exercise Physiology: People and Ideas*: Oxford University Press; 2003; p. 255-91.
[33] Fitts RH. Cellular mechanisms of muscle fatigue. *Physiol Rev*, 1994, 74, 49-94.
[34] Bassett DR, Jr., Howley ET. Limiting factors for maximum oxygen uptake and determinants of endurance performance. *Med Sci Sports Exerc*, 2000, 32, 70-84.
[35] Bassett DR, Jr. Scientific contributions of A. V. Hill: exercise physiology pioneer. *J Appl Physiol*, 2002, 93, 1567-82.
[36] Howley ET. VO2 max and the plateau - needed or not? *Med Sci Sports Exerc*, 2007, 39, 101-2.
[37] Noakes TD. Testing for maximum oxygen consumption has produced a brainless model of human exercise performance. *Br J Sports Med*, 2008, 42, 551-5.
[38] Tucker R, Rauch L, Harley YX, Noakes TD. Impaired exercise performance in the heat is associated with an anticipatory reduction in skeletal muscle recruitment. *Pflugers Arch*, 2004, 448, 422-30.
[39] Tucker R, Marle T, Lambert EV, Noakes TD. The rate of heat storage mediates an anticipatory reduction in exercise intensity during cycling at a fixed rating of perceived exertion. *J Physiol*, 2006, 574, 905-15.
[40] Bigland-Ritchie B, Rice CL, Garland SJ, Walsh ML. Task-dependent factors in fatigue of human voluntary contractions. *Adv Exp Med Biol*, 1995, 384, 361-80.
[41] Gandevia SC. Spinal and supraspinal factors in human muscle fatigue. *Physiol Rev*, 2001, 81, 1725-89.
[42] Noakes TD. The central governor model of exercise regulation applied to the marathon. *Sports Med*, 2007, 37, 374-7.
[43] Tucker R, Lambert MI, Noakes TD. An analysis of pacing strategies during men's world record performances in track athletics. *Int J Sports Physiol Per*, 2006, 1, 233-45.
[44] Noakes TD, Lambert M, Human R. Which lap is the slowest? An analysis of 32 world record performances. *Br J Sports Med*, 2008.
[45] Tucker R, Bester A, Lambert EV, Noakes TD, Vaughan CL, St Clair GA. Non-random fluctuations in power output during self-paced exercise. *Br J Sports Med*, 2006, 40, 912-7.
[46] Liebenberg L. Persistence hunting by modern hunter-gatherers. *Curr Anthrop*, 2006, 47, 1017-25.
[47] Liebenberg L. The relevance of persistence hunting to human evolution. *J Hum Evol*, 2008, 55, 1156-9.
[48] Lieberman DE, Bramble DM. The evolution of marathon running : capabilities in humans. *Sports Med*, 2007, 37, 288-90.

[49] Amann M, Eldridge MW, Lovering AT, Stickland MK, Pegelow DF, Dempsey JA. Arterial oxygenation influences central motor output and exercise performance via effects on peripheral locomotor muscle fatigue in humans. *J Physiol*, 2006, 575, 937-52.

[50] Noakes TD, Marino FE. Arterial oxygenation, central motor output and exercise performance in humans. *J Physiol*, 2007, 585, 919-21.

[51] Baisch K. Fall von chronischem tetanus. *Deutsche MedWehnschr*, 1917, 42, 1624-6.

[52] Wilhelm T. La cyphose tétanique. *J Chir*, 1923, 22, 295.

[53] Roberg OT. Spinal deformity following tetanus and its relation to juvenile kyphosis. *J Bone Joint Surg*, 1937, 19, 603-29.

[54] Polatin P, Friedman MM, Harris MM, Horwitz WA. Vertebral fractures produced by metrazol-induced convulsions. *J Am Med Assoc*, 1939, 112, 1684-7.

[55] Bennett BT, Fitzpatrick CP. Fractures of the spine complicating metrazol therapy. *J Am Med Assoc*, 1939, 112, 2240-4.

[56] Hamsa WR, Bennett AE. Traumatic complications of convulsive shock therapy. *J Am Med Assoc*, 1939, 112, 2244-6.

[57] Swart J, Lamberts RP, Lambert MI, St Clair GA, Lambert EV, Skowno J, et al. Exercising with reserve: evidence that the central nervous system regulates prolonged exercise performance. *Br J Sports Med*, 2009, 43, 782-8.

[58] Borg G. *Borg's Perceived Exertion and Pain Scales*. Champaign, IL: Human Kinetics; 1998.

[59] Noakes TD. Rating of perceived exertion as a predictor of the duration of exercise that remains until exhaustion. *Br J Sports Med*, 2008, 42, 623-4.

[60] Baldwin J, Snow RJ, Gibala MJ, Garnham A, Howarth K, Febbraio MA. Glycogen availability does not affect the TCA cycle or TAN pools during prolonged, fatiguing exercise. *J Appl Physiol*, 2003, 94, 2181-7.

[61] Noakes TD. Linear relationship between the perception of effort and the duration of constant load exercise that remains. *J Appl Physiol*, 2004, 96, 1571-2.

[62] Crewe H, Tucker R, Noakes TD. The rate of increase in rating of perceived exertion predicts the duration of exercise to fatigue at a fixed power output in different environmental conditions. *Eur J Appl Physiol*, 2008, 103, 569-77.

[63] Trojian TH, Beedie CJ. Placebo effect and athletes. *Curr Sports Med Rep*, 2008, 7, 214-7.

[64] Beedie CJ, Stuart EM, Coleman DA, Foad AJ. Placebo effects of caffeine on cycling performance. *Med Sci Sports Exerc*, 2006, 38, 2159-64.

[65] Foad AJ, Beedie CJ, Coleman DA. Pharmacological and psychological effects of caffeine ingestion in 40-km cycling performance. *Med Sci Sports Exerc*, 2008, 40, 158-65.

[66] Beedie CJ, Coleman DA, Foad AJ. Positive and negative placebo effects resulting from the deceptive administration of an ergogenic aid. *Int J Sport Nutr Exerc Metab*, 2007, 17, 259-69.

[67] Barwood MJ, Weston NJV, Thelwell R, Page J. A motivational music and video intervention improves high-intensity exercise performance. *J Sports Sci Med*, 2009, 8, 422-42.

[68] Lim HB, Atkinson G, Karageorghis CI, Eubank MR. Effects of differentiated music on cycling time trial. *Int J Sports Med*, 2009, 30, 435-42.

[69] Chambers ES, Bridge MW, Jones DA. Carbohydrate sensing in the human mouth: effects on exercise performance and brain activity. *J Physiol*, 2009, 587, 1779-94.
[70] Roelands B, Hasegawa H, Watson P, Piacentini MF, Buyse L, De SG, et al. Performance and thermoregulatory effects of chronic bupropion administration in the heat. *Eur J Appl Physiol*, 2009, 105, 493-8.
[71] Marcora SM, Staiano W, Manning V. Mental fatigue impairs physical performance in humans. *J Appl Physiol*, 2009, 106, 857-64.
[72] Micklewright D, Papadopoulou E, Swart J, Noakes T. Previous experience influences pacing during 20 km time trial cycling. *Br J Sports Med*, 2010.
[73] Morton RH. Deception by manipulating the clock calibration influences cycle ergometer endurance time in males. *J Sci Med Sport*, 2009, 12, 332-7.
[74] Mauger AR, Jones AM, Williams CA. Influence of feedback and prior experience on pacing during a 4-km cycle time trial. *Med Sci Sports Exerc*, 2009, 41, 451-8.
[75] Wittekind AL, Micklewright D, Beneke R. Teleoanticipation in all-out short duration cycling. *Br J Sports Med*, 2009.
[76] Seifert T, Rasmussen P, Secher NH, Nielsen HB. Cerebral oxygenation decreases during exercise in humans with beta-adrenergic blockade. *Acta Phil*, 2009, 196, 295-302.
[77] Rasmussen P, Nybo L, Volianitis S, Moller K, Secher NH, Gjedde A. Cerebral oxygenation is reduced during hyperthermic exercise in humans. *Acta Phil*, 2010.
[78] Thomas R, Stephane P. Prefrontal cortex oxygenation and neuromuscular responses to exhaustive exercise. *Eur J Appl Physiol*, 2008, 102, 153-63.
[79] Rasmussen P, Nielsen J, Overgaard M, Krogh-Madsen R, Gjedde A, Secher NH, et al. Reduced muscle activation during exercise related to brain oxygenation and metabolism in humans. *J Physiol*, 2010, [in press].
[80] Tucker R. The anticipatory regulation of performance: the physiological basis for pacing strategies and the development of a perception-based model for exercise performance. *Br J Sports Med*, 2009, 43, 392-400.
[81] Ansley L, Robson PJ, St Clair GA, Noakes TD. Anticipatory pacing strategies during supramaximal exercise lasting longer than 30 s. *Med Sci Sports Exerc*, 2004, 36, 309-14.
[82] Ansley L, Schabort E, St Clair GA, Lambert MI, Noakes TD. Regulation of pacing strategies during successive 4-km time trials. *Med Sci Sports Exerc*, 2004, 36, 1819-25.
[83] Tucker R, Noakes TD. The physiological regulation of pacing strategy during exercise: a critical review. *Br J Sports Med*, 2009, 43, e1.
[84] Castle PC, Macdonald AL, Philp A, Webborn A, Watt PW, Maxwell NS. Precooling leg muscle improves intermittent sprint exercise performance in hot, humid conditions. *J Appl Physiol*, 2006, 100, 1377-84.
[85] Joseph T, Johnson B, Battista RA, Wright G, Dodge C, Porcari JP, et al. Perception of fatigue during simulated competition. *Med Sci Sports Exerc*, 2008, 40, 381-6.
[86] Marino FE, Lambert MI, Noakes TD. Superior performance of African runners in warm humid but not in cool environmental conditions. *J Appl Physiol*, 2004, 96, 124-30.
[87] Marino FE. Anticipatory regulation and avoidance of catastrophe during exercise-induced hyperthermia. *Comp Biochem Physiol B Biochem Mol Biol*, 2004, 139, 561-9.

[88] Albertus Y. Critical analysis of techniques for normalising electromyographic data. Cape Town: University of Cape Town; 2008.

[89] Noakes TD. Evidence that reduced skeletal muscle recruitment explains the lactate paradox during exercise at high altitude. *J Appl Physiol*, 2009, 106, 737-8.

[90] Marcora SM, Staiano W. The limit to exercise tolerance in humans: mind over muscle? *Eur J Appl Physiol*, 2010.

[91] Kay D, Marino FE, Cannon J, St Clair GA, Lambert MI, Noakes TD. Evidence for neuromuscular fatigue during high-intensity cycling in warm, humid conditions. *Eur J Appl Physiol*, 2001, 84, 115-21.

[92] Eston R, Faulkner J, St Clair GA, Noakes T, Parfitt G. The effect of antecedent fatiguing activity on the relationship between perceived exertion and physiological activity during a constant load exercise task. *Psychophysiology*, 2007, 44, 779-86.

[93] Altareki N, Drust B, Atkinson G, Cable T, Gregson W. Effects of environmental heat stress (35 degrees C) with simulated air movement on the thermoregulatory responses during a 4-km cycling time trial. *Int J Sports Med*, 2009, 30, 9-15.

[94] Flouris AD, Cheung SS. Human conscious response to thermal input is adjusted to changes in mean body temperature. *Br J Sports Med*, 2009, 43, 199-203.

[95] Morante SM, Brotherhood JR. Autonomic and behavioural thermoregulation in tennis. *Br J Sports Med*, 2008, 42, 679-85.

[96] Noakes TD, Calbet JA, Boushel R, Sondergaard H, Radegran G, Wagner PD, et al. Central regulation of skeletal muscle recruitment explains the reduced maximal cardiac output during exercise in hypoxia. *American Journal of Physiology-Regulatory Integrative and Comparative Physiology*, 2004, 287, R996-R9.

[97] Johnson BD, Joseph T, Wright G, Battista RA, Dodge C, Balweg A, et al. Rapidity of responding to a hypoxic challenge during exercise. *Eur J Appl Physiol*, 2009, 106, 493-9.

[98] Clark SA, Bourdon PC, Schmidt W, Singh B, Cable G, Onus KJ, et al. The effect of acute simulated moderate altitude on power, performance and pacing strategies in well-trained cyclists. *Eur J Appl Physiol*, 2007, 102, 45-55.

[99] Tucker R, Kayser B, Rae E, Raunch L, Bosch A, Noakes T. Hyperoxia improves 20 km cycling time trial performance by increasing muscle activation levels while perceived exertion stays the same. *Eur J Appl Physiol*, 2007, 101, 771-81.

[100] Edwards AM, Mann ME, Marfell-Jones MJ, Rankin DM, Noakes TD, Shillington DP. The influence of moderate dehydration on soccer performance: physiological responses to 45-min of outdoors match-play and the immediate subsequent performance of sport-specific and mental concentration tests. *Br J Sports Med*, 2007, 41, 385-91.

[101] Rauch HG, St Clair Gibson A, Lambert EV, Noakes TD. A signalling role for muscle glycogen in the regulation of pace during prolonged exercise. *Br J Sports Med*, 2005, 39, 34-8.

[102] Lima-Silva A, Pires FO, Bertuzzi RCM, Lira FS, Casarini D, Kiss MA. Low carbohydrate diet affects the oxygen uptake on kinetics and rating of perceived exertion in high intensity exercise. *Psychophysiology*, 2010, (in press).

[103] Racinais S, Bringard A, Puchaux K, Noakes TD, Perrey S. Modulation in voluntary neural drive in relation to muscle soreness. *Eur J Appl Physiol*, 2007.

[104] Marcora SM, Bosio A. Effect of exercise-induced muscle damage on endurance running performance in humans. *Scand J Med Sci Sports*, 2007, 17, 662-71.

[105] Baron B, Deruelle F, Moullan F, Dalleau G, Verkindt C, Noakes TD. The eccentric muscle loading influences the pacing strategies during repeated downhill sprint intervals. *Eur J Appl Physiol*, 2009, 105, 749-57.

[106] Bean WB, Eichna LW. Performance in relation to environmental temperature. *FedProc*, 1943, 144-58.

[107] Bannister RG. Muscular effort. *Br Med Bull*, 1956, 12, 222-5.

[108] Entine J. *Taboo: Why black athletes dominate sports and why we're afraid to talk about it*. New York: Public Affairs; 2000.

[109] Noakes TD, St Clair Gibson A, Lambert EV. From catastrophe to complexity: a novel model of integrative central neural regulation of effort and fatigue during exercise in humans: summary and conclusions. *Br J Sports Med*, 2005, 39, 120-4.

[110] Noakes TD, St Clair Gibson A, Lambert EV. From catastrophe to complexity: a novel model of integrative central neural regulation of effort and fatigue during exercise in humans. *Br J Sports Med*, 2004, 38, 511-4.

In: Regulation of Fatigue in Exercise
Editor: Frank E. Marino

ISBN 978-1-61209-334-5

Chapter 2

Two-way Interactions between Mental and Physical Stressors and their Role in Fatigue

Stephen S. Cheung*
Environmental Ergonomics Laboratory, Department of Physical Education and Kinesiology, Brock University, 500 Glenridge Avenue, St. Catharines, Ontario, L2S-3A1, Canada

Abstract

Exercise capacity is dependent on many factors, with multiple triggers proposed for the onset of fatigue. One model for exercise regulation is from a behavioural or psychological perspective, where the organism integrates input from a variety of internal and external cues to derive a conscious decision on an efficient or optimal level of effort while avoiding catastrophic physiological collapse. If the brain is a strong controller or integrator for exercise, then it appears logical that significant stress on the brain, whether it be physiological, neurohumoral or biochemical changes [1], or mental from high cognitive effort, should influence exercise capacity. This chapter will examine the two-way interactions between high levels of mental stress and exercise-induced fatigue. It will also explore whether motor skills or cognitive functioning can be preserved in the face of extreme physiological fatigue, and their implications to sports and occupational training.

Introduction

It is indisputable that "fatigue," defined here as a decrease in voluntary or involuntary exercise capacity, occurs with sustained exercise. This is a common occurrence in endurance sports requiring sustained submaximal repetitions such as running, cycling, or swimming, and

* 905-688-5550x5662 (w); 905-688-8364 (f); stephen.cheung@brocku.ca

a number of theoretical models have been proposed to contribute to such development of fatigue in both thermoneutral [2] and hot [3] environments. It is also common consensus in athletic settings that physiological fatigue elicits impairment in skilled sports (e.g. racquet) requiring both repetitive movements and tactical decision making [4, 5]. Indeed, the interaction between physical and mental fatigue is implicit and paramount in sports, as much of training and strategy revolves around degrading an opponent's mental and motor skills through pushing them to the point of physical fatigue. The difficulty is understanding what happens physiologically as that point of fatigue approaches and what factors contribute to determining exercise capacity and tolerance [6], especially as the primary factors may vary depending on sport, individual characteristics such as fitness and training status, and environmental issues such as temperature and altitude.

One recent paradigm in understanding exercise capacity is the interaction between peripheral factors and centrally-regulated determination of voluntary effort. Rather than the traditional view that exercise is limited by failure in one or more physiological systems (e.g. metabolic, cardiovascular, muscular), voluntary exercise is proposed to start and end in the brain [7]. Within this framework, the brain is proposed to integrate a wide range of physiological inputs in an anticipatory or feed-forward fashion, with the end goal of maintaining optimal or maximal exercise capacity while avoiding catastrophic failure of any system or the body as a whole [8-10]. One interesting dimension to the discussion concerning the relative contributions of the brain versus the peripheral muscles to exercise fatigue, but which has largely been ignored to date by physiologists, has come from investigations into the effects of mental activity on exercise, and vice versa. If the brain is a strong controller or integrator for exercise, then it appears logical that significant stress on the brain, whether it be physiological [11], neurohumoral or biochemical changes [1] or mental from high cognitive effort [12], should influence exercise capacity. Examples of this interaction include diminished levels of arousal, as assessed by EEGs, upon the attainment of voluntary exhaustion in the heat [13, 14], and also in higher subjective ratings of perceived exertion and altered brain activity in the heat despite no changes in electromyographic activity [13]. Similarly, the physiological stress stemming from exercise should also impact cognitive function and mental task performance.

The purpose of this review, therefore, is to explore the interactions between mental activity and exercise capacity. The focus will be on whether significant mental stress can influence exercise capacity and the reverse of whether exercise influences cognitive functioning and mental performance. Finally, we will also explore whether motor skills or cognitive functioning can be preserved in the face of extreme physiological or mental fatigue, and their implications to sports and occupational training [15].

Mental Activity and Exercise

Surprisingly, while the effects of exercise or environmental stressors on cerebral physiology [1, 15, 16], along with investigations on the effects of exercise on mood and mental health [17, 18], have been a heavy field of research within the past decades, data on whether mental activity impairs exercise performance has been almost completely missing until very recently [19]. In contrast, the bulk of data on mental stress effects on exercise has come indirectly from studies on the etiology and diagnosis of overreaching, overtraining and burnout [20, 21]. In such reports, high levels of psychosocial stress related to personal or competitive issues is assumed to be a contributor to the lower performance levels that remains the main criterion for defining overtraining. This is a different question than the effects of direct and acute mental stress on performance, along with the confounding effects from the wide range of immunological and neurohumoral changes associated with overtraining. Therefore, this section will focus on the few studies available where exercise is performed during or following heavy mental efforts.

In healthy, non-overtrained subjects, strong experimental evidence linking mental fatigue to reduced exercise performance was recently provided by Marcora et al. [12]. In this experimental protocol, 90 min of a cognitively demanding vigilance task was employed to elicit mental fatigue compared to 90 min viewing of a neutral television commentary. Subsequent tolerance times during a ride to exhaustion at 80% of their peak power output was significantly shorter following the mental task (640 ± 316 s) than with neutral (754 ± 339 s) conditions. Importantly, self-reported motivation levels were not different following the two mental manipulations, yet subjective sensations of fatigue were higher before the exercise task. This higher sensation of effort and fatigue carried over into the actual exercise, where ratings of perceived exertion were significantly higher following the mental task despite no differences in the physiological responses over time. Overall, the data suggests that elevated strain in cognitive functioning negatively impacted exercise capacity through mental rather than physiological pathways, though the linking mechanism integrating mental effort and physical capacity remains unexplored.

A threshold effect of mental stress may be evident, such that mental stress might need sufficient intensity to significantly stress the overall human system before it will begin impairing exercise performance. Indeed, mild mental stimulation may actually contribute to improved physiological response to exercise, analogous to the well-documented effect of crowds or psychological stimuli improving performance of skilled tasks [22]. When a moderately stressful vigilance task requiring continuous attention and pattern recognition was performed during a soccer-simulation treadmill run, heart rates were lower [23]. Importantly, this lower physiological strain occurred without change in the actual treadmill protocol and therefore externally-imposed stress, nor in the level of blood lactate, salivary cortisol and only mild changes in ratings of perceived exertion. Overall, while no direct cognitive measures were taken, the authors proposed that the improved physiological response may be attributed to enhancing dissociation and diverting attention from the treadmill run. If dissociation or a change to external focus is a mechanism for improvement in physiological responses, an unexplored avenue appears to be the potentially different effects of this distractor in people with preference for internal versus external psychological focus [24].

SUMMARY

In summary, only minimal direct information is available on the effects of acute mental stress immediately prior to or concurrent with exercise in healthy subjects, leaving the field ripe for further research. Future avenues include whether there is a threshold or an optimal level of mental stress to enhance exercise capacity. This meshes with demonstration by

Barwood et al. [25-27] that psychological training improved exercise capacity in the heat and also prolonged breath-hold times in cold water, such that the physiological bases for sport psychology may become more closely examined and quantified.

Exercise Effects on Cognition

Mood, feelings of energy and fatigue, along with mental health can be improved by exercise [18], and this is typically explicitly or implicitly suggested as one of the many health benefits from increasing physical activity in the general population. Much of the work on synergies between mental stress and exercise has come from the field of psychology, where exercise is used as an experimental manipulation to elicit physiological stress or fatigue, and cognitive function becomes the primary test of interest. Namely, does exercise improve mental performance, or can mild to heavy exercise blunt or otherwise impair cognitive functioning? This interaction is typically one of the implied goals of increasing fitness in a sporting context, where fatigue is often blamed for poor decision making. Similarly, in occupational health and safety, fatigue from physical or environmental stress may be responsible for increasing the risks of cognitive impairment and accidents [28, 29]. Overall, evidence for exercise-induced impairment of mental functioning is equivocal, and the focus of this section will be on the effects of exercise-induced fatigue on mental and task performance in a sporting context.

Impaired Cognition

A body of evidence suggests that moderate exercise can significantly degrade components of the information processing pathway ranging from simple cognitive response through to complex decision making. Yagi et al. [30] employed the common experimental psychology technique of analyzing the P300 event-related potential waveform in response to auditory or visual "oddball" stimuli. With cycling exercise at a moderate intensity of 130-150 bpm, the latency of the P300 wave decreased, typically representative of a faster rate of cognitive processing. However, the amplitude of the wave decreased, indicative of a diminished attentional resource allocated to the stimulus. Complementary data to these cognitive findings were reported in actual performance measures. Reaction time – a combination of both cognitive and motor performance, decreased during exercise when responding to either visual or auditory stimuli. However, the error rate also increased during exercise. Overall, the authors concluded that exercise resulted in a faster but weaker cognitive response to external stimulus.

These data are supported with intermittent and variable treadmill running simulating a 90-min soccer match, where response time to the vigilance task gradually improved over the course of exercise but the accuracy degraded [23]. One extrapolation from such data is that athletes may make faster but inappropriate decisions as exercise or matches progressed. Furthermore, such accuracy errors may possibly increase the risk of injury, such as from not recognizing and properly evading collisions. Further support for a negative effect of exercise on cognitive function comes from research into higher-level complex executive functioning.

In performing a random number generation task, subjects adopted less effortful and complex strategies with the onset of moderate aerobic cycling, which was maintained throughout exercise; however, complexity returned to baseline levels immediately upon termination of exercise [31].

The above mental impairment from exercise can be interpreted with a holistic framework of the human organism having a baseline or preferred capacity to compensate for overall stressors to the system, as outlined by Robert and Hockey [32]. In this model, an interactive two-stage control of overall performance is achieved through continuous analysis of "effort" leading to compensatory control of mental resource allocation. Therefore, with an increase in stress, greater allocation of resources would result in greater perceived mental or physiological effort. Alternately, overall perceived effort and mental resources may be preserved by adopting lower performance goals or less complex strategies. While primarily derived from behavioural psychology, such a model appears readily adaptable to an exercise context, where enhanced physiological strain forms an additional input to the body's overall integration of effort or stress [33]. In turn, decreasing cognitive functioning or complexity of responses by the individual serves to minimize the overall demands on mental resource allocation during exercise [31]. Such a model of exercise and environmental stress [34] also readily accommodates the observations of greater subjective ratings of perceived effort with exercise following mental stress [12], decreased mental arousal with hyperthermia [14], and a perceptual underestimation of physiological strain during heat stress with increased fitness and theoretically greater physiological reserve [35].

Preserved Cognition

Opposing a major role for exercise fatigue on cognitive functioning, a series of studies from a French research group has found that, in general, reaction times to a mental task improved without significant impairment in accuracy. Reaction times to a pattern recognition task with different levels of stimulus degradation along with response options were progressively faster at 20% and 50% of maximal aerobic power cycling exercise, with elevated mental arousal and catecholaminergic stimulation proposed as possible mechanisms for improved response times [36]. Similarly, response time (time from stimulus onset to initiation of a motor response) decreased consistently by 10-15 ms throughout the entire continuum of overall response times with no impairment in either the variability of response or accuracy with a choice (two-hand by two direction) reaction time task when performed at 90% of ventilatory threshold power [37].

One limitation of reaction time studies is that reaction by itself can be a "black box" that makes it difficult to separate the various components of a complete response, ranging from cognitive processing of the stimulus through to motor coordination to affect an appropriate response. Some data suggest that exercise actually has minimal effect on cognitive performance, but rather that improvement comes from enhanced motor facilitation. Davranche et al. [38] found, in athletes involved in decision-making sports (e.g. team, racquet, fighting sports), that reaction times to both weak and strong intensity signals with a visual pattern recognition task were shortened during exercise. However, electromyographic data on the thumb used to respond to the stimulus demonstrated that the pre-motor reaction time was in fact not altered by exercise, but rather that the improvement can be attributed to a faster motor phase; furthermore, similar motor time improvements occurred with both weak and strong signal intensity [38, 39]. Further EMG analysis indicated that the facilitation could be attributed to an improved synchronization of motor unit discharge [38], suggesting that exercise may have a priming effect on enhancing overall coordination even with movements not directly related to the exercise. However, the potential mechanism behind exercise benefits on motor functioning, especially on improved motor patterning, remain unclear and open to further research [40].

While of high scientific fidelity, the ecological validity of cognitive tasks isolating particular components of the information processing pathway can make extrapolation to actual exercise and sporting situations problematic. Royal et al. [41] attempted to comprehensively investigate the effects of incrementally greater fatigue on various components of team sports performance. In a group of junior elite male water polo players, intermittent but maximal effort 20-s swimming/shooting drills with progressively less recovery between repetitions (80 down to 10 s) elicited a wide variety of effects on sports performance. The stronger fatigue sets, not surprisingly, elicited higher heart rates, ratings of perceived exertion, lactate levels, and also a degradation in the biomechanical proficiency involved in penalty shooting. However, the higher levels of fatigue, against hypothesis, actually improved the accuracy of decision making on a water polo-specific tactical test. Overall preservation of sports performance was maintained despite the disparate findings in its foundational components, in that no effect was observed on penalty shooting velocity or accuracy. It is unclear why the decision making was improved with greater physiological strain, as this contrasts with the general views, summarized above, of a faster but less accurate decision with fatigue [30]. One possibility is that the highly-experienced athletes may have been accustomed and more highly aroused by the realism of the sport-specific exercise and test in this particular study. In contrast, the generalized fatigue from non-specific exercise such as cycling or treadmill exercise, along with non-specific and non-familiar cognitive and performance tasks, may have elicited lower levels of arousal or motivation in subjects in other studies [41].

Complementing cognitive and performance tasks, one advance over the past decade has been the increasing utilization of transcranial magnetic stimulation (TMS) to monitor activity at the level of the motor cortex in response to exercise or environmental stressors. TMS appears highly sensitive to the particular muscles being employed with a particular exercise task, as Tergau et al. [42] observed that intracortical facilitation significantly decreased only in the active (brachioradialis) versus non-active (aductor pollicis) muscles following a pull-up to exhaustion task. In coordination with electroencephalographic or neuro-imaging data, TMS may thus aid in mapping the neural responses to exercise, or in isolating the location at which fatigue occurs. For example, Todd et al. [43] reported that increased cortical activity remained possible with moderate passive hyperthermia that did not elicit muscular fatigue, but that this enhanced central activity remained unable to compensate for impaired muscle properties from hyperthermia, resulting in an overall decrement in voluntary force that likely occurs at a level below the motor cortex.

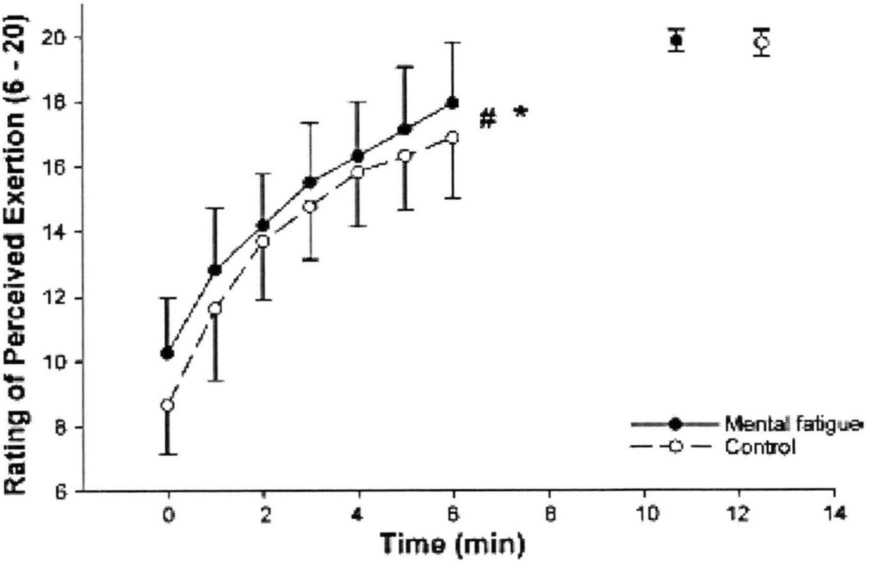

Figure 1. Mental fatigue from 90 min of a highly-demanding cognitive task resulted in a consistently higher subjective perception of effort throughout cycling to exhaustion at a constant workload of 80% of peak power output. Voluntary tolerance time also significantly decreased by 15% compared to following a neutral mental task, with maximal perceived effort at exhaustion in both conditions. (Reprinted from [12] Used with permission).

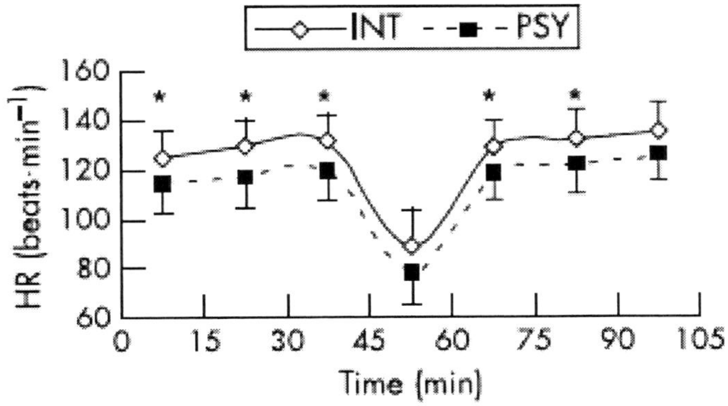

Figure 2. Heart rate responses to a 90 minute soccer-simulation treadmill run, performed either with no cognitive task or while performing a vigilance task. Heart rate was significantly lower throughout all 15 min segments except for the final segment, despite the exercise intensity being identical and externally paced in both conditions. No differences were observed in blood lactate or salivary cortisol responses between conditions, with ratings of perceived exertion lower during the second 15 minute segment of the first half during the vigilance task. (From [23] Used with permission).

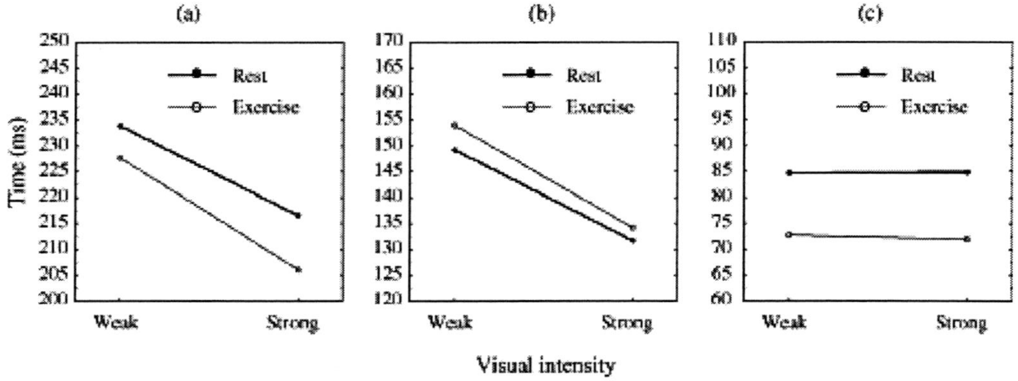

Figure 3. Electromyographic analysis demonstrates that the improvement in overall reaction time with increasing exercise at both weak and strong stimulus (left figure) was not due to acceleration of the cognitive, pre-motor phase (middle figure), but was due to a systematic enhancement of the motor phase of response (right figure). (From [38]. Used with permission).

SUMMARY

The effects of exercise and increased physiological strain on cognitive functioning and mental performance remains unclear. Part of the uncertainty revolves around the wide gamut that constitutes task performance, from informational processing and non-motor aspects along with movement planning and execution, through to neuromuscular activity and feedback. This is exacerbated by the body's apparent ability to compensate for minor impairments within individual components along the entire pathway. Therefore, one of the key avenues for research in the coming years appears to be a better understanding of how to properly and comprehensively quantify cognitive performance changes in an exercising context.

PRESERVATION OF PERFORMANCE

A third approach to investigating the interaction between mental and physical performance is to pose the question: "Are there basic mental and/or motor skills that are so ingrained that they are resistant to "fatigue" from hard exercise?" From an evolutionary perspective, it would seem logical that humans would never have survived our early days of "hunt and be hunted" if we were not able to function and perform essential survival skills while chasing prey (e.g. throwing a spear) or being chased by hungry and toothy critters (e.g. simple motor coordination in running across rough terrain). Can relatively modern and novel skills be learned and ingrained to be resistant to fatigue from hard exercise? A research group from Hong Kong recently investigated this question in a pair of studies [44, 45], utilizing the underhanded rugby pass as the novel skill. This particular task appears a reasonable choice, as it's not inherently as natural as a single-armed overhand throw used with a spear, rock, or baseball. Naïve subjects learned the skill via either an implicit (errorless) or an explicit (errorful) protocol, then performed the test before and after two Wingate sprints [45] to elicit anaerobic fatigue or a ramp VO_{2max} test [44] to elicit aerobic fatigue. Compared to control subjects with no learning of the skills, accuracy in the rugby pass test was much higher with both styles of learning before and after the exercise manipulation. However, implicit learning, where minimal errors were made over the course of learning, was more resistant to exercise-induced fatigue in both studies [44, 45].

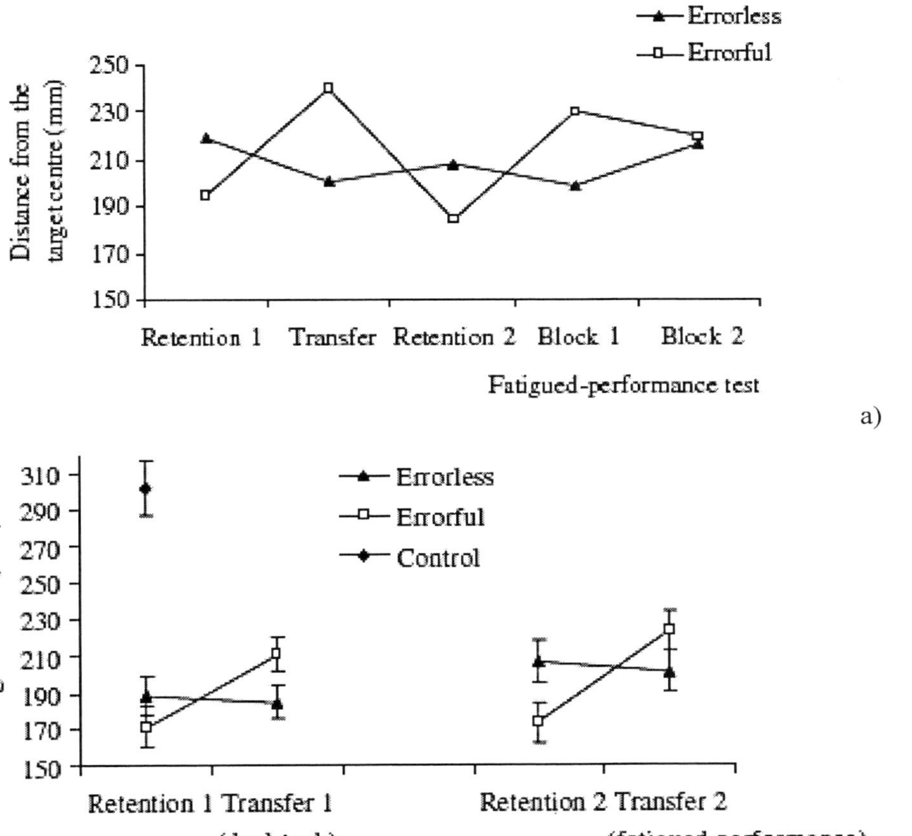

Figure 4. a) Two Wingate anaerobic sprints had minimal impact on underhanded rugby toss accuracy (blocks 1 and 2), although some degradation was observed when the toss was taught using an explicit, errorful instructional method (retention 2 was the final pre-trial test, compared to Block 1 as the first ten tosses following exercise). b) Accuracy results following maximal aerobic exercise with both implicit, errorless instruction versus explicit, errorful instruction. Accuracy was retained both following initial learning of the task (transfer 1) and also following a year with no further exposure to the skill (transfer 2), with both significantly better than a control group with no training. (From [45, 44]. Used with permission)

Interestingly, accuracy was essentially maintained at initial post-learning levels when the test was repeated with and without exercise following a year with no further experience in rugby passing [45]. This demonstrates that both learning processes were successful in training and retaining a novel skill and well-learned skills seem very resistant to extreme fatigue. In terms of the interaction between mental and peripheral factors during exercise fatigue, this ability to ingrain skills to the point of becoming "instinctive" or habitual suggests that motor output, in some instances, can be separated from central or peripheral fatigue induced by either exercise or likely strong mental stress. Again, the mechanism underlying this long term learning and motor patterning remains unknown. This has also been reported with motor skills such as the synchronization of grasping and grip force modulation despite the decay of sensory input from local hand cooling or removal of visual input [46]. Specifically, the force used to grasp the object was consistently higher throughout the lifting task, but the pattern of that force modulation remained similar with either hand cooling or blinding. It is proposed that a centrally-controlled feedforward pattern anticipated the force and coordination required to perform the task, making it resistant to peripheral impairment of the hand and also to central strain from mild heating or cooling of core temperature [46].

SUMMARY

Findings of skill retention despite exercise fatigue is of course important from an athletic perspective, as much of sports training and strategy revolves around degrading an opponent's mental and motor skills through pushing them to the point of physical fatigue. Arguably, it is even more crucial in occupational settings, where proper training of emergency responses can make the difference between life and death. For example, with offshore petroleum installation heavily reliant on helicopter transport for its personnel, periodic retraining of emergency escape skills from a ditched helicopter is required. However, determining the frequency of such training recertification is tempered by the loss in time and productivity. Therefore, understanding the nature and mechanisms underlying retention of such skills with different training programs become essential in establishing the best ways to train and retain such skills under the extreme mental and physical stress involved in actual emergency situations.

CONCLUSION

The discussion on the synergies between mental and physical stressors demonstrate the strong capacity of the central nervous system in modulating or overriding peripheral control of sports performance and vice versa. The nature and mechanisms underlying such interactions remain largely unexplored despite the critical role decision making and mental stress has in safe and successful athletic and occupational exercise. Furthermore, the additional stress caused by environmental stressors such as extreme temperatures or altitude may compound mental or physiological stress, further contributing to a degradation of performance or acceleration of fatigue [34]. With advances in technology and measurement capabilities such as neuroimaging and transcranial magnetic stimulation, future research will hopefully seek a closer integration of psychological and physiological responses to exercise and environmental extremes.

REFERENCES

[1] Meeusen R, Watson P, Hasegawa H, Roelands B, Piacentini MF. Central fatigue: The serotonin hypothesis and beyond. *Sports Med*, 2006, 36, 881-909.

[2] Abbiss CR, Laursen PB. Models to explain fatigue during prolonged endurance cycling. *Sports Med*, 2005, 35, 865-98.

[3] Cheung SS, Sleivert GG. Multiple triggers for hyperthermic fatigue and exhaustion. *Exerc Sport Sci Rev*, 2004, 32, 100-6.

[4] Davey PR, Thorpe RD, Williams C. Fatigue decreases skilled tennis performance. *J Sports Sci*, 2002, 20, 311-8.

[5] Hornery DJ, Farrow D, Mujika I, Young W. Fatigue in tennis: Mechanisms of fatigue and effect on performance. *Sports Med*, 2007, 37, 199-212.

[6] Hargreaves M. Fatigue mechanisms determining exercise performance: Integrative physiology is systems biology. *J Appl Physiol*, 2008, 104, 1541-2.

[7] Kayser B. Exercise starts and ends in the brain. *Eur J Appl Physiol*, 2003, 90, 411-9.

[8] Lambert EV, St Clair Gibson A, Noakes TD. Complex systems model of fatigue: Integrative homoeostatic control of peripheral physiological systems during exercise in humans. *Br J Sports Med*, 2005, 39, 52-62.

[9] Noakes TD, St Clair Gibson A, Lambert EV. From catastrophe to complexity: A novel model of integrative central neural regulation of effort and fatigue during exercise in humans: summary and conclusions. *Br J Sports Med*, 2005, 39, 120-4.

[10] St Clair Gibson A, Goedecke JH, Harley YX, Myers LJ, Lambert MI, Noakes TD, et al. Metabolic setpoint control mechanisms in different physiological systems at rest and during exercise. *J Theor Biol*, 2005, 236, 60-72.

[11] Nybo L. Hyperthermia and fatigue. *J Appl Physiol*, 2008, 104, 871-8.

[12] Marcora SM, Staiano W, Manning V. Mental fatigue impairs physical performance in humans. *J Appl Physiol*, 2009, 106, 857-64.

[13] Nybo L, Nielsen B. Perceived exertion is associated with an altered brain activity during exercise with progressive hyperthermia. *J Appl Physiol*, 2001, 91, 2017-23.

[14] Nielsen B, Hyldig T, Bidstrup F, Gonzalez-Alonso J, Christoffersen GRJ. Brain activity and fatigue during prolonged exercise in the heat. *Pflügers Archive: European Journal of Physiology*, 2001, 442, 41-8.

[15] Nybo L. Exercise and heat stress: Cerebral challenges and consequences. *Prog Brain Res*, 2007, 162, 29-43.

[16] Davis J, Bailey SP. Possible mechanisms of central nervous system fatigue during exercise. *Med Sci Sports Exerc*, 1997, 29, 45-57.

[17] Peluso MA, Guerra de Andrade LH. Physical activity and mental health: The association between exercise and mood. *Clinics*, 2005, 60, 61-70.

[18] Puetz TW, O'Connor PJ, Dishman RK. Effects of chronic exercise on feelings of energy and fatigue: A quantitative synthesis. *Psychol Bull*, 2006, 132, 866-76.

[19] Cheung SS. Neuropsychological determinants of exercise tolerance in the heat. *Prog Brain Res*, 2007, 162, 45-60.

[20] Anish EJ. Exercise and its effects on the central nervous system. *Curr Sports Med Rep*, 2005, 4, 18-23.

[21] Halson SL, Jeukendrup AE. Does overtraining exist?: An analysis of overreaching and overtraining research. *Sports Med*, 2004, 34, 967-81.
[22] Strauss B. Social facilitation in motor tasks: A review of research and theory. *Psych Sport Exerc*, 2002, 3, 237-56.
[23] Greig M, Marchant D, Lovell R, Clough P, McNaughton L. A continuous mental task decreases the physiological response to soccer-specific intermittent exercise. *Br J Sports Med*, 2007, 41, 908-13.
[24] Weiner B. Attribution, emotion, and action. In: Sorrentino RM, Higgins ET, editors. *Handbook of Motivation and Cognition: foundations of social behavior*. New York: Guilford Press; 1986; p. 281-312.
[25] Barwood MJ, Dalzell J, Datta AK, Thelwell RC, Tipton MJ. Breath-hold performance during cold water immersion: Effects of psychological skills training. *Aviat Space Environ Med*, 2006, 77, 1136-42.
[26] Barwood MJ, Datta AK, Thelwell RC, Tipton MJ. Breath-hold time during cold water immersion: Effects of habituation with psychological training. *Aviat Space Environ Med*, 2007, 78, 1029-34.
[27] Barwood MJ, Thelwell RC, Tipton MJ. Psychological skills training improves exercise performance in the heat. *Med Sci Sports Exerc*, 2008, 40, 387-96.
[28] Hancock PA, Vasmatzidis I. Effects of heat stress on cognitive performance: The current state of knowledge. *Int J Hyperthermia*, 2003, 19, 355-72.
[29] Pilcher JJ, Nadler E, Busch C. Effects of hot and cold temperature exposure on performance: A meta-analytic review. *Ergo*, 2002, 45, 682-98.
[30] Yagi Y, Coburn KL, Estes KM, Arruda JE. Effects of aerobic exercise and gender on visual and auditory P300, reaction time, and accuracy. *Eur J Appl Physiol Occup Physiol*, 1999, 80, 402-8.
[31] Audiffren M, Tomporowski PD, Zagrodnik J. Acute aerobic exercise and information processing: Modulation of executive control in a Random Number Generation task. *Acta Psychol (Amst)*, 2009, 132, 85-95.
[32] Robert G, Hockey J. Compensatory control in the regulation of human performance under stress and high workload: A cognitive-energetical framework. *Biol Psychol*, 1997, 45, 73-93.
[33] Craig AD. How do you feel? Interoception: The sense of the physiological condition of the body. *Nat Rev Neurosci*, 2002, 3, 655-66.
[34] Paulus MP, Potterat EG, Taylor MK, Van Orden KF, Bauman J, Momen N, et al. A neuroscience approach to optimizing brain resources for human performance in extreme environments. *Neurosci Biobehav Rev*, 2009, 33, 1080-8.
[35] Tikuisis P, Mclellan TM, Selkirk G. Perceptual versus physiological heat strain during exercise-heat stress. *Med Sci Sports Exerc*, 2002, 34, 1454-61.
[36] Davranche K, Audiffren M. Facilitating effects of exercise on information processing. *J Sports Sci*, 2004, 22, 419-28.
[37] Davranche K, Audiffren M, Denjean A. A distributional analysis of the effect of physical exercise on a choice reaction time task. *J Sports Sci*, 2006, 24, 323-9.
[38] Davranche K, Burle B, Audiffren M, Hasbroucq T. Physical exercise facilitates motor processes in simple reaction time performance: An electromyographic analysis. *Neurosci Lett*, 2006, 396, 54-6.

[39] Davranche K, Burle B, Audiffren M, Hasbroucq T. Information processing during physical exercise: A chronometric and electromyographic study. *Exp Brain Res*, 2005, 165, 532-40.

[40] Davranche K, McMorris T. Specific effects of acute moderate exercise on cognitive control. *Brain Cogn*, 2009, 69, 565-70.

[41] Royal KA, Farrow D, Mujika I, Halson SL, Pyne D, Abernethy B. The effects of fatigue on decision making and shooting skill performance in water polo players. *J Sports Sci*, 2006, 24, 807-15.

[42] Tergau F, Geese R, Bauer A, Baur S, Paulus W, Reimers CD. Motor cortex fatigue in sports measured by transcranial magnetic double stimulation. *Med Sci Sports Exerc*, 2000, 32, 1942-8.

[43] Todd G, Butler JE, Taylor JL, Gandevia SC. Hyperthermia: A failure of the motor cortex and the muscle. *J Physiol (Lond)*, 2005, 563, 621-31.

[44] Masters RS, Poolton JM, Maxwell JP. Stable implicit motor processes despite aerobic locomotor fatigue. *Conscious Cogn*, 2008, 17, 335-8.

[45] Poolton JM, Masters RS, Maxwell JP. Passing thoughts on the evolutionary stability of implicit motor behaviour: Performance retention under physiological fatigue. *Conscious Cogn*, 2007, 16, 456-68.

[46] Cheung SS, Reynolds LF, Macdonald MA, Tweedie CL, Urquhart RL, Westwood DA. Effects of local and core body temperature on grip force modulation during movement-induced load force fluctuations. *Eur J Appl Physiol*, 2008, 103, 59-69.

In: Regulation of Fatigue in Exercise
Editor: Frank E. Marino

ISBN 978-1-61209-334-5

Chapter 3

METABOLIC ACIDOSIS AND FATIGUE: WHERE TO FROM HERE?

***R. A. Robergs*[1,*], *D. Kennedy*[2]**
[1]Exercise Physiology and Biochemistry, Exercise Physiology Laboratories, Exercise Science Program, The University of New Mexico, Albuquerque, NM 87131-1258, USA
[2] Paradigm Physical Therapy & Wellness, Albuquerque, NM, USA

ABSTRACT

For the last 35 years the central focus of acidosis has been on lactic acid or lactate as being the cause of acidosis and acidosis being the cause of fatigue during intense exercise. Unfortunately, causation has been implied from correlation. The organic chemistry of the lactate dehydrogenase reaction clearly demonstrates the error of the development of metabolic acidosis from lactate production. This is not to detract from the significant development of acidosis during intense exercise. However, the assumed negative effect of acidosis on contractile failure is also called into question. The purpose of this review and commentary is to reflect on past research that has investigated the role of acidosis in fatigue, provide extensive evidence from the record of prior and current ^{31}P MRS research on muscle acidosis during exercise and recovery and provide further insight into proton balance during muscle energy catabolism based on computations of multiple competing cation and pH-dependent proton stoichiometry. Finally, we suggest the role of acidosis in fatigue may have a greater effect outside of the cell.

INTRODUCTION

For more than 100 years, the development of metabolic acidosis has been heralded as a major contributor to the fatigue accompanying intense exercise and therefore a determinant of intense sports and athletic performance. Such a belief has also been connected to the misconception of the production of lactic acid in contracting skeletal muscle and the

* Phone: (505) 277-2658; Email: rrobergs@unm.edu

consequent lactic acidosis. We now know that exercise-induced metabolic acidosis is not caused by lactate production [1], that there is a negligible presence of lactic acid in human tissue, and that the biochemical explanation of metabolic acidosis is far more complex than the concept of all blame being given to one molecule; lactic acid. Nevertheless, it is important to once again recognize the irrefutable facts of the organic chemistry of the lactate dehydrogenase reaction, as shown in Figure 1.

The reduction of pyruvate to lactate involves the metabolic buffering of 1 proton (H^+) per lactate formation, and this stoichiometry is remarkably constant across the physiological muscle pH range (6.1 to 7.0) (Figure 1) with proton coefficients of 0.9897 and 0.9938, respectively. Lactate production also regenerates NAD^+, and as such is an important, if not essential feature of the metabolic characteristic of sustained ATP turnover from glycolytically fueled muscle contraction (Figure 2). In other words, without lactate production, glycolytic ATP regeneration and muscle contractile function during intense exercise would be severely compromised.

Table 1. Muscle and blood pH measurements during intense whole body or regional exercise in humans*

Model	Muscle pH	Method	Blood pH	Ref
Human Whole Body				
Intermittent intense running or cycling (vastus lateralis)	6.41	Biopsy homogenate pH electrode	6.94 (capillary samples)	28
Intense cycling (vastus lateralis)	6.6	Biopsy homogenate pH electrode		60
400 m sprint running (gastrocnemius)	6.63	Biopsy homogenate pH electrode	7.1 (venous)	14
Human Regional				
Knee extension – vastus lateralis	6.74	^{31}P MRS		71
Knee extension – vastus lateralis	6.77	Biopsy homogenate pH electrode		71
Knee extension – vastus lateralis	6.54	^{31}P MRS		63
Dynamic forearm wrist flexion	6.52	^{31}P MRS		53
Knee extension – vastus lateralis (electrical stimulation)	6.43	Biopsy homogenate pH electrode		66
Isometric knee extension – vastus lateralis (occluded circulation)	6.56	Biopsy homogenate pH electrode		59
Isometric wrist flexion	6.42	^{31}P MRS		45
Isometric wrist flexion	6.24	^{31}P MRS		2
Finger flexion	6.55	^{31}P MRS		58

* Not intended to be a thorough representation of published research.

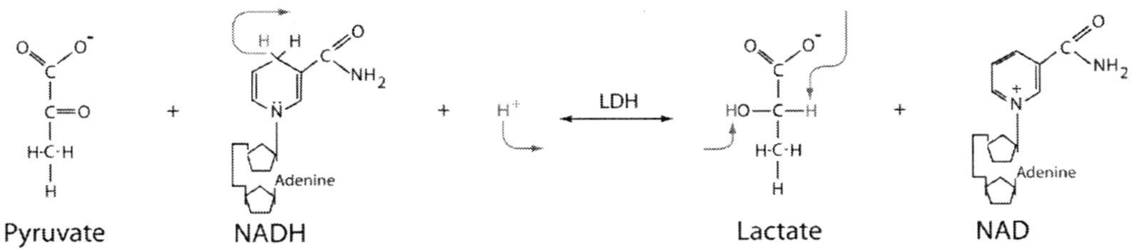

Figure 1. The lactate dehydrogenase reaction, showing proton (H^+) metabolic buffering and NAD^+ regeneration for glycolysis. The carboxylic acid functional group of pyruvate and lactate remain deprotonated as they are never produced in their acid form and remain so due to the low pKa of 2.26 and 3.67, respectively.

The absence of lactic acid and misconception of a lactic acidosis does not detract from the fact that skeletal muscle and the systemic circulation can develop extreme acidosis during intense exercise. Data from ^{31}P MRS has quantified muscle pH to decrease from 7.0 to 6.2 during repeated short term intense muscle contractions to volitional exhaustion [2]. In addition, venous blood pH decreases from 7.4 to as low 7.15 (mixed venous) have been documented for sustained intense cycle ergometry exercise to volitional failure [3] (Table 1). Blood and muscle acidosis can be sustained for at least 30 min during passive recovery, and for some individuals is also accompanied with severe nausea [3, 4]. Juel et al. [5-8] and others [9] have quantified the exercise training responses of the monocarboxylate lactate and proton transporter in skeletal muscle, thereby revealing the importance of proton and lactate efflux from muscle to blood (Figure 2) and the contribution of the proton load of intense muscle contraction to systemic metabolic acidosis.

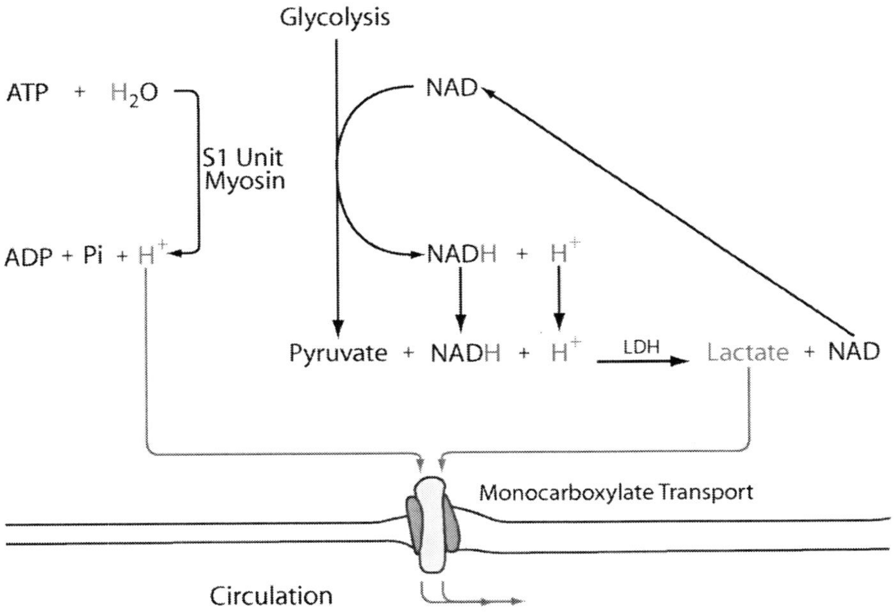

Figure 2. The combined transport of lactate and a proton (H^+) from muscle to blood as a support of continued glycolytic ATP turnover during intense exercise.

Several reviews have been written on the topic of lactate and/or acidosis and muscle fatigue in recent years [10-12]. Consequently, the purpose of this review and commentary is to reflect on past research that has investigated the role of acidosis in fatigue, provide extensive evidence from the record of prior ^{31}P MRS research on muscle acidosis during exercise and recovery, present some of our recent, as yet unpublished ^{31}P MRS findings, and provide further insight into proton balance during muscle energy catabolism based on computations of multiple competing cation and pH-dependent proton stoichiometry. Final discussion will then be given ON the need to combine knowledge of physico-chemical buffering to computations of proton release from energy catabolism to improve understanding of the biochemistry of exercise-induced metabolic acidosis. Knowing the biochemistry of metabolic acidosis, in combination with implications of acidosis to muscle fatigue, will enable scientists to ask and answer the question, "Where to from here?"

Research Methods Used to Study Acidosis and Fatigue

A variety of methods have been used to research the potential influence of acidosis on muscle fatigue during intense exercise, and these methods are summarized in Figure 3. Brief overviews of this research and their contributions to revealing the potential impact of acidosis to the fatigue of intense exercise are provided in separate sections below.

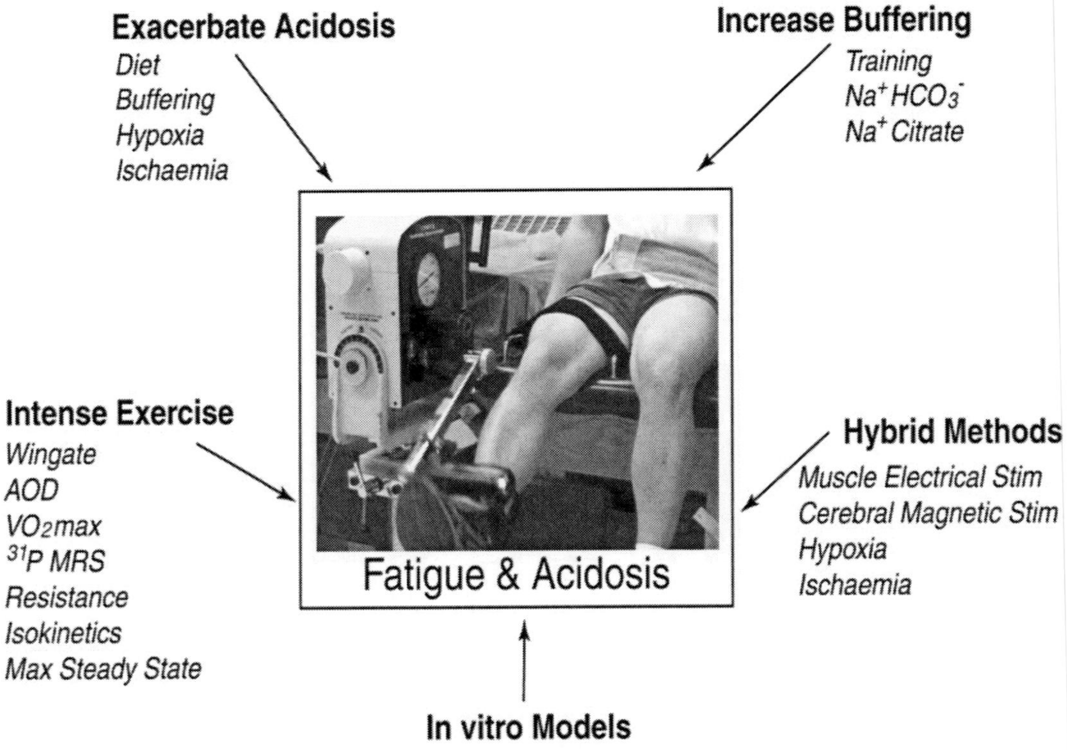

Figure 3. Summary of methods used to study exercise-induced metabolic acidosis and fatigue.

Intense Exercise and Metabolic Acidosis

It is beneficial to understand the historical development of the evidence of exercise-induced metabolic acidosis, as well as the extent of metabolic acidosis documented from various human experimental exercise conditions and in vitro muscle models from various animal species. A summary of these findings is presented in Table 1. Intense exercise has the capability to lower muscle pH to values between 6.0 to 6.8, with this pH range revealing considerable variability in end-exercise muscle pH. The lowest muscle pH data come from research using magnetic resonance techniques. Research of the metabolic acidosis of intense exercise has always assumed that the acidosis is a negative occurrence to muscle energetic and/or contractile function. For example, the classic research, though not necessarily correctly interpreted, Sahlin et al. [13-15] demonstrated that muscle pH decreased to 6.4 following high intensity isometric exercise, and that such decreases correlated highly (r=0.96) to the accumulation of muscle lactate and pyruvate (Figure 4a). Interestingly, in the same study by Sahlin et al. [14] a similar correlation was presented between muscle pH and a log transformation of a version of what has become known as the phosphorylation potential (log ([creatine] [ATP] / [creatine phosphate] [ADP]) for muscle in response to different conditions of intense sustained or intermittent isometric exercise (Figure 4b). A decrease in the phosphorylation potential is interpreted as increased non-steady state metabolic stress in contracting muscle, or in other words, a condition of ATP demand exceeding ATP supply from glycolysis and mitochondrial respiration. Interestingly, Sahlin's correlation presentation of acidosis and the phosphorylation potential never received the attention and acknowledgement as the correlation of pH to lactate + pyruvate. Presumably, the concept of metabolic acids causing acidosis was more in-line with scientific thought at that time [16].

A summary of this research is very clear. Intense exercise induces a severe metabolic acidosis. Muscle pH can fall as much as 1 pH unit, and blood pH can fall as much as 0.45 pH units depending on where blood is sampled from relative to the exercising muscle mass. Metabolic acidosis also coincides with the accumulation of glycolytic intermediates and lactate, which remain good predictors of alterations in muscle acid-base balance.

Exacerbating the Acidosis of Intense Exercise

If methods that exacerbate acidosis increase fatigue or decrease exercise performance, such results provide indirect evidence for the detriment of metabolic acidosis to muscle metabolism and/or systemic physiology during exercise. There are few studies that have followed this line of inquiry from a nutrition perspective. Nevertheless, Robergs et al. [4] compared placebo (pH=7.16) to nutritional alkalosis (0.2 g/kg $Na^+HCO_3^-$ + 0.2 g/kg Na^+citrate; pH=7.21) or acidosis (0.3 g/kg NH_4Cl; pH=7.15) and showed that pre-exercise acidosis resulted in significantly shorter time to fatigue when cycling at 110% Watts@VO_2max compared to both placebo and alkalosis.

Exercise at increased altitude has been more widely applied to study exacerbated acidosis and exercise performance. Exposure to the hypoxia of higher altitude induces an acute and chronic decrease in blood bicarbonate due to a sustained hypoxic hyperventilation and commensurate respiratory alkalosis. As such, an early rationale for studying exercise at altitude was that the hypoxia and associated decreased blood buffering capacity, despite a resting respiratory alkalosis, would exacerbate the development of metabolic acidosis. Such rationale was proven incorrect by Adams et al. [17] who revealed higher end exercise blood pH during hypoxia ($FIO_2 = 0.12$) than normoxia.

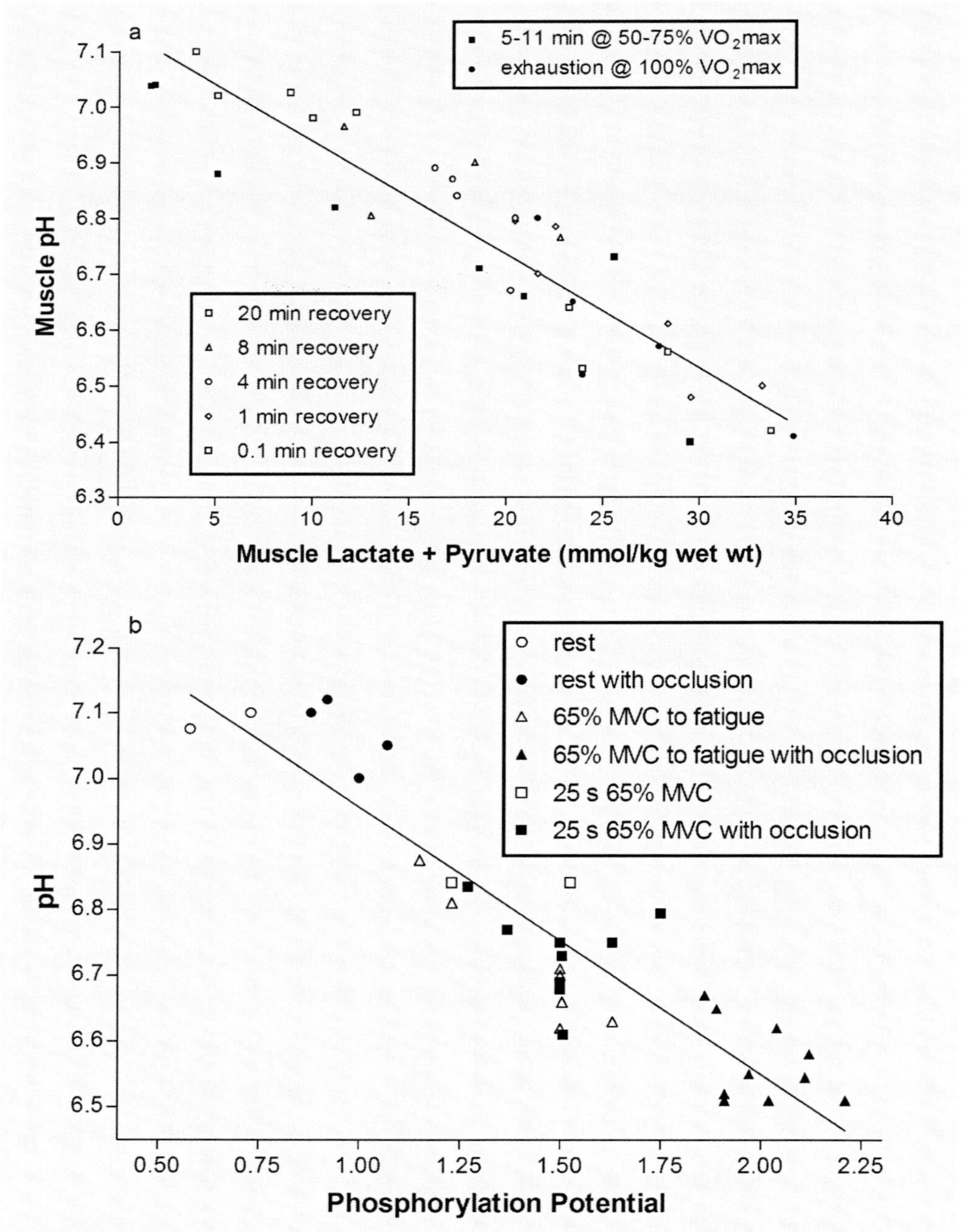

Figure 4. Early research of the change in muscle pH for different rest, exercise and recovery conditions and the association of muscle pH to pyruvate, lactate and the cytosolic phosphorylation potential (log(([creatine][ATP]) / ([creatine phosphate][ADP])). Adapted from Sahlin et al. (59,60).

Hogen et al. [18] used ^{31}P MRS to study the muscle (gastrocnemius) phosphagen system in six subjects during incremental plantar flexion exercise exposed to graded hypoxia (FIO_2 = 0.1), normoxia (FIO_2 = 0.21), or hyperoxia (FIO_2 = 1.0). The exercise-induced decrease in muscle pH had a significantly earlier onset and more rapid change in the hypoxia condition. End-exercise muscle pH was not different between conditions; 6.84, 6.9 and 6.92, respectively. However, it is interesting that the pH values were not lower compared to other ^{31}P MRS investigations (see Table 1), and that such non-significant findings are difficult to interpret due to the low sample size and marginally adequate statistical power (d=0.8, α = 0.05, 1-β = 0.85, n = 6; GPower 3.1, Universität Kiel, Germany). The final data interpretations were that regardless of oxygen availability, exercise is terminated when intracellular conditions develop that are no longer commensurate with continued muscle contraction. The intracellular conditions reported across all trials were a mild acidosis, which is not revealing of a role of acidosis to end exercise, and more importantly, similar relative changes (compared to rest) in muscle [CrP] (~42%) and increased [Pi] (~440%). These metabolic similarities occurred despite significant differences in time to exhaustion between FIO_2 conditions.

There are clearly more complex issues involved in exercise to exhaustion than a decrease in muscle or systemic pH.

Decreasing the Acidosis of Intense Exercise

Normal Ionic Exchange during Exercise

During rest conditions, acid-base balance in muscle is primarily maintained by Na^+/H^+ transport in conjunction with Na^+/bicarbonate co-transport. Na^+ is brought into the cell in exchange for H^+ in both systems, however this creates an increased intracellular [Na^+], which requires remediation by the Na^+/K^+ pump. With increased Na^+/K^+ pump activity, increased energy demand occurs, which can ultimately constrain Na^+/H^+ exchange and bicarbonate co-transport for effective buffering and pH maintenance during intense exercise [7]. In addition, considerable K^+ efflux from muscle raises interstitial [K^+], which can impair the membrane potential and contribute to electrophysiological contributions to muscle fatigue [19-21].

During high intensity exercise pH regulation is better mediated by lactate/H^+ co-transport. Increasing H^+ from ATP turnover and glycolysis during intense exercise coincides with, but is not stoichiometric with, lactate production and accumulation. The release of lactate and H^+ from the cell has also been shown to occur at similar rates [22], though others have provided evidence that such stoichiometry is larger for H^+ efflux [7-9]. The export of lactate and H^+ ions into the interstitium, vascular system, and mitochondria is mediated by the monocarboxylate transporters (MCT1 and MCT4) and can account for 70-75% of the efflux of H^+ out of the cell to offset the rapid decline of intracellular pH [9]. The MCT system transport of H^+ out of the cell allows the H^+ to be buffered in the interstitium and vascular system via HCO_3^- in the carbonic anhydrase reaction [9]. Additionally, the MCT1 is found in the mitochondrial membrane suggesting that the mitochondria might also provide a H^+ buffering mechanism and additional mitochondrial derived metabolic clearance of lactate [23, 24].

Exercise Training

Improvements in proton buffering can be attained through quality training. Intermittent, high intensity training has been shown to increase the density of MCTs and Na^+/H^+ transport proteins (by as much as 15%), which will increase H^+ export from the cell and improve pH regulation [8]. Another mechanism that may account for improved H^+ release with training is an improved capillary density. With increased blood flow to the working muscle smaller muscle-to-arterial concentration gradients exist creating improved buffering via HCO_3^- [7]. Training also increases cellular protein through classic hypertrophy, thereby increasing structural H^+ buffering. Furthermore, training increases the capacity of the phosphagen system, and because of the improved MCT facilitated efflux of lactate, increases the capacity of lactate production. Reactions of the phosphagen system and lactate production represent the muscle cell's largest contributors to metabolic H^+ buffering.

Ingestion of Buffering Agents

Ingestion of sodium citrate prior to an intense exercise bout can also improve acid-base regulation. Acute ingestion of sodium citrate has been shown to reduce post exercise acidosis following intense exercise [4, 25]. However, improved exercise performance with sodium citrate ingestion has not been established. In several studies the ingestion of sodium citrate, while improved acid-base balance was demonstrated, exercise performance during Wingate testing, or exercise to exhaustion at 95% ,100%, and 110% VO_{2max} failed to demonstrate improved exercise capacity [4, 25-27].

The ingestion of sodium bicarbonate ($Na^+HCO_3^-$) was first investigated some 80 years ago and at that time was found to have some ergonomic benefit [28]. Further work in the 1970's and 1980's continued to find that the use of $Na^+HCO_3^-$ could be beneficial to exercise performance [29]. The use of $Na^+HCO_3^-$ to improve high intensity exercise has been more recently demonstrated during competitive cycle ergometry. This improvement is thought to derive from improved buffering capacity and maintenance of resting levels of pH through a 60 min bout [30]. Similarly, a study using ^{31}P MRS during incremental forearm exercise to exhaustion found a 12% improvement in peak power with ingestion of $Na^+HCO_3^-$ [31].

Overall, the ingestion of $Na^+HCO_3^-$ appears to have a potentially beneficial effect on performance for both long-term and short-term high-intensity exercise, and more so for intense intermittent exercise [32, 33]. The mechanism of improved performance from establishing pre-exercise alkalosis seems unclear, though it would appear that any ergogenic effect would depend on the exercise condition creating an acid-base disequilibrium. Nevertheless, evidence also exists to show that pre-exercise alkalosis may benefit muscle from a deceased K+ efflux [20].

HYBRID METHODS

The main hybrid method that we will mention here pertains to electrical stimulation of human muscle accompanied by muscle biopsy and biochemical assay of metabolites. Such a design is beneficial because artificial stimulation removes the role of the central nervous system from fatigue and the decision to end exercise, thereby possibly revealing more complete muscle biochemical contributions to fatigue. Spriet et al. [34] have done classic research of this type. Seven male subjects received electrical stimulation of the antero-lateral thigh involving 1.6 s stimulation followed by 1.6 s recovery. Subjects were stimulated to perform 64 contractions during complete anoxia induced by a thigh cuff inflated to 250 mmHg. Muscle biopsies were taken from the vastus lateralis at rest, and in the recovery interval following 16 and 48 contractions. The contralateral leg was then prepared and underwent similar testing, except muscle biopsies occurred in the recovery intervals after 32 and 64 contractions. Muscle biopsies were prepared for and assayed for glycolytic intermediates, lactate and pH (homogenate technique). Ironically, despite such involuntary and arguably supra-maximal contractions, muscle pH did not decrease below 6.43. Such intramuscular conditions coincided with a 40% decrease in muscle ATP.

As with all research based on muscle biopsy, the low temporal resolution of the muscle sampling, in combination with the delays inherent in sampling and possible errors of the homogenate technique, muscle pH data are inherently high compared to results from ^{31}P MRS (see Table 1). While validation work of muscle pH from ^{31}P MRS to biopsy (homogenate) methods has revealed an acceptable validity coefficient (r=0.88) [35], the pH range studied in this investigation was narrow (7.14 to 6.77) thereby limiting the external validity of these findings.

In-Vitro Methods

Early *in vitro* studies of muscle fibers demonstrated that a low pH was detrimental to muscle performance resulting in reduced force production and shortening velocity [36-41]. This early work was initially linked to lactic acid as the source of acidification of the cell, though this construct has since been repudiated [1]. Still, several mechanisms were identified including enzyme inhibition, particularly of phosphofructokinase, interference with Ca^{++} regulation at the sarcoplasmic reticulum, disruption of cross-bridge cycling, and slowed relaxation time.

pH Effects on Enzymes

Initial in vitro studies suggested decreasing pH to have an inhibitory effect on phosphorylase and PFK [41]. However, subsequent investigation, particularly of in vivo or in situ muscle calls this finding into question. Using in situ methods of rat muscle at physiologic temperature, increasing acidification failed to inhibit PFK and phosphorylase activity, allowing continued ATP regeneration by glycolysis [42]. In humans, changes in PFK activity have been shown to remain unchanged during acidic conditions based on observation of continued gylcogenolysis [43-45].

Force Generation/Velocity

With declination of intra- and extracellular pH, decreased contractile force and velocity of contraction have been demonstrated by in vitro work with tissue samples at 25°C [39, 40].

The loss of force was thought to arise from both interference of Ca^{++} binding at troponin C through competition of H^+ at the binding site, thus slowing cross-bridge detachment, and H^+ interference with Ca^{++} release from the SR due to a charge differential across the membrane. However, subsequent investigation at higher temperatures demonstrated decreased affects of acidosis on fatigue. Pate et al [46] and Westerblad et al [47] found that acidification at 30°C and 32°C decreased peak force 18% and 10% respectively. This was a significant change from the 53% and 28% drop in peak force found at lower temperatures [46, 47]. It should be noted in these studies that the drop in peak force was for maximum tetanic contraction, which is not reflective of in vivo intrinsic muscle performance. More recently, Knuth et al [48] also found that loss of peak force was improved from 30% at 15°C to 11% at 30°C at a pH of 6.2.

Decreased contraction velocity due to a reduction in cross-bridge detachment rate in the presence of increased [H^+] has shown similar improvement with increasing temperature and appears to be dependent more on increasing [Pi] than a low pH [49]. While there appears to be a slight effect of acidification on force generation/velocity, this effect has not been examined at actual muscle physiologic temperatures (due to methodology constraints) or at equivalent in vivo muscle contraction conditions. It is possible that at higher temperatures the effect of acidosis on force generation/velocity may be even smaller.

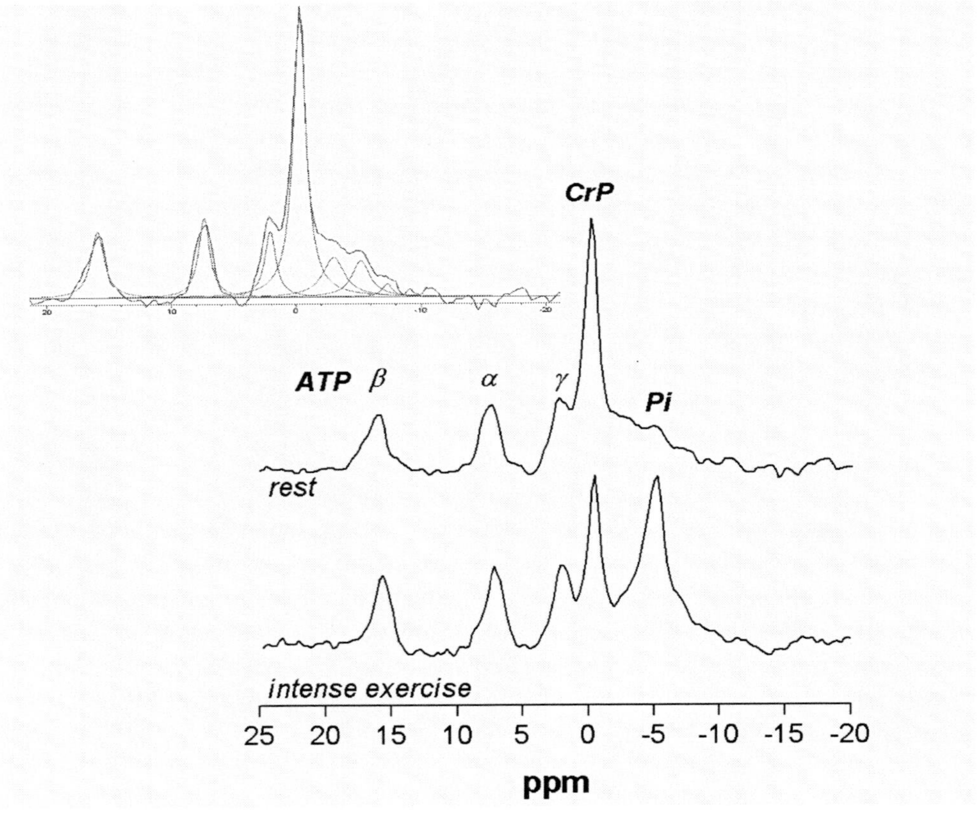

Figure 5. Spectra from ^{31}P MRS for the medial gastrocnemius at rest and after intense exercise. The upper left image shows data processing involving Lorentzian curve fitting of the rest condition spectrum.

The upper insert of Figure 5 presents the same rest spectrum after line fitting with Lorentzian curves. The area under each curve is proportional to metabolite concentration, and typically the muscle ATP concentration of 8.2 mmol/kg wet wt is assigned to the □ATP phosphate peak, and then used as an internal standard to calculate the remaining phosphate metabolites [51]. The respective concentrations for Pi and CrP based on this method for this spectrum are 6.0 and 32.0 mmol/kg wet wt.

The effects of acidification are further complicated by research on single fiber preparations demonstrating that acidification of the fiber maintained or improved force generation [50]. Increased $[K^+]$ was found to decrease muscle force production due to changes in membrane potential and reduction in action potential (AP) propagation down the T system resulting in decreased Ca^{++} release from the SR. But under acidic conditions, this effect was remediated by decreased Cl^- permeability and reduction of the AP threshold, therefore allowing greater AP propagation and force generation [19]. Thus under conditions where the AP propagation rate may lead to fatigue, a low pH may help preserve muscle function and delay the onset of fatigue.

In summary, establishing more physiologic conditions of in vitro research, particularly with respect to temperature, has changed the understanding of low pH on muscle fatigue; it now appears that a low pH has a far less inhibitory effect on contractile function and in certain circumstances may act to preserve muscle activation thus offsetting any detrimental effects leading to force reduction.

CONTRIBUTIONS OF ^{31}P MRS TO THE STUDY OF EXERCISE-INDUCED METABOLIC ACIDOSIS

The method of ^{31}P MRS has enormous capabilities for the study of muscle metabolic acidosis. Figure 5 presents a ^{31}P spectrum acquired from the medial gastrocnemius of a 48 year old female subject. All peaks are labeled, and note that the resonance frequency of phosphate groups differs slightly depending on their neighboring atomic conditions. The x-axis unit ppm is an adjustment of the resonance frequency (MHz) based on the magnetic field strength of the magnet. This normalizes the signals and thereby enables spectra from different magnets to be compared.

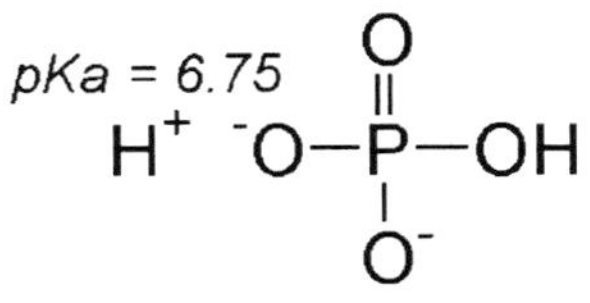

Figure 6. The chemical structure of inorganic phosphate. One of the ionizable oxygen atoms has a pKa within the physiological pH range. As muscle pH falls below 7, a greater proportion of inorganic phosphate molecules becomes protonated. As such, muscle inorganic phosphate functions as a proton (H^+) buffer within skeletal muscle.

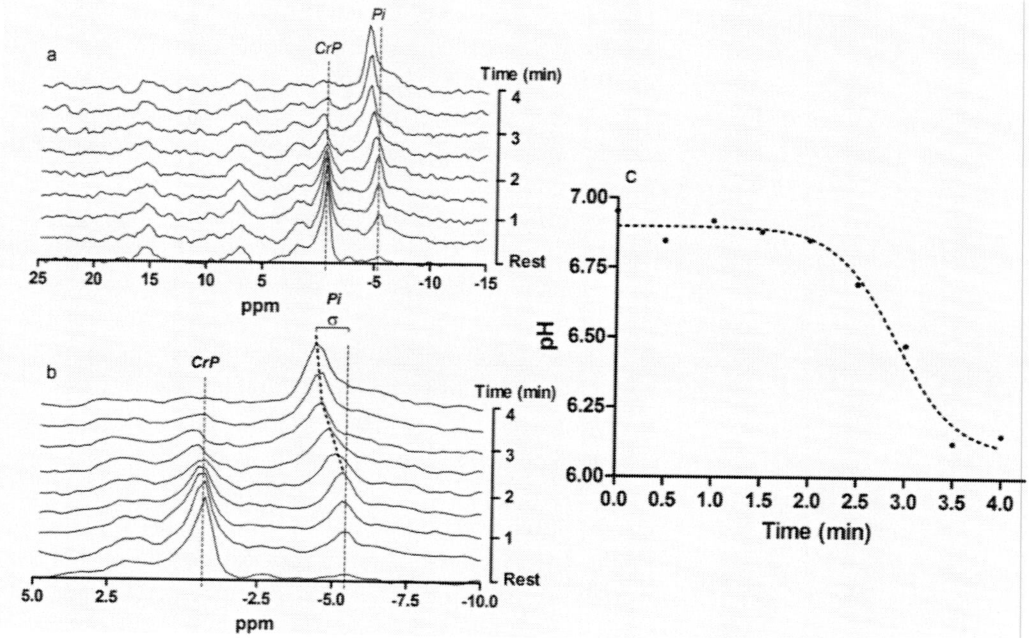

Figure 7. a) Stacked spectra from ^{31}P MRS for the combined Palmaris Longus and Flexor Carpi Radialis muscles of the forearm at rest and after 1 min stages (1 kg increment) of incremental wrist flexion exercise. b) The same data of a) focused to the resonance range from creatine phosphate (Cr) to inorganic phosphate (Pi). The shift in resonance frequency of Pi (δ) is shown by the dashed lines. c) The computed pH for the individual spectra.

The resonance frequency (ppm) difference between Pi and CrP is pH dependent. As muscle pH falls, a larger proportion of Pi molecules acquire a proton to the sole ionizable oxygen across the physiological range of pH (Figure 6). This protonation alters the resonance frequency of the phosphate group, causing the Pi peak to migrate closer to the CrP of the ^{31}P spectrum. A spectrum for the gastrocemius acquired during intense plantar flexion exercise is presented in the bottom image of Figure 5. Muscle pH is calculated from ^{31}P spectra using a modification of the Henderson-Hasselbach equation (Equation 1). For the spectra of Figure 5, muscle pH had decreased from 7.0 at rest to 6.82 during repeated intense plantar flexion contractions.

$$pH = 6.75 + \log_{10} [\delta - 3.350 / (5.6 - \delta]$$ Equation 1

The quality of ^{31}P spectra is proportional to the volume of the sampled muscle and the magnetic field strength. The spectra presented in Figure 5 is from a 1.8 Tesla magnet (1 Tesla = 1,000 gauss = 3,000 x earth's equatorial magnetic field strength of 0.3 gauss). Higher field strength magnets allow greater resolution between phosphate peaks and increased temporal resolution. For example, the spectra of Figure 1 represent 1 min of data, resulting from the sum of 12 spectra where each was acquired every 5 s. A 3 Tesla magnet provides greater signal to noise, and thereby allows for the summation of fewer spectra, with quality data obtainable in time intervals as short as 10 s [51, 52].

The research and scientific benefit of using ^{31}P MRS to study muscle pH changes is based on the non-invasive nature and high temporal resolution of the method. Intramuscular pH measurements that can occur in frequent time intervals enable quantification of the kinetic response of pH change during and in recovery from intense exercise. For example, Figure 7 presents the ^{31}P MRS spectra obtained from dynamic forearm wrist flexion exercise for one subject in another of our recent investigations. This subject was able to fully tax his phosphagen system, diminishing the CrP signal to within the noise of the spectra of Figure 7a and b. The shift in resonance frequency of Pi between minutes 2 and 4 is clearly seen in Figure 7b. Intramuscular pH decreased rapidly during the third and fourth stages of this protocol, attaining peak acidosis of pH = 6.12 (Figure 7c).

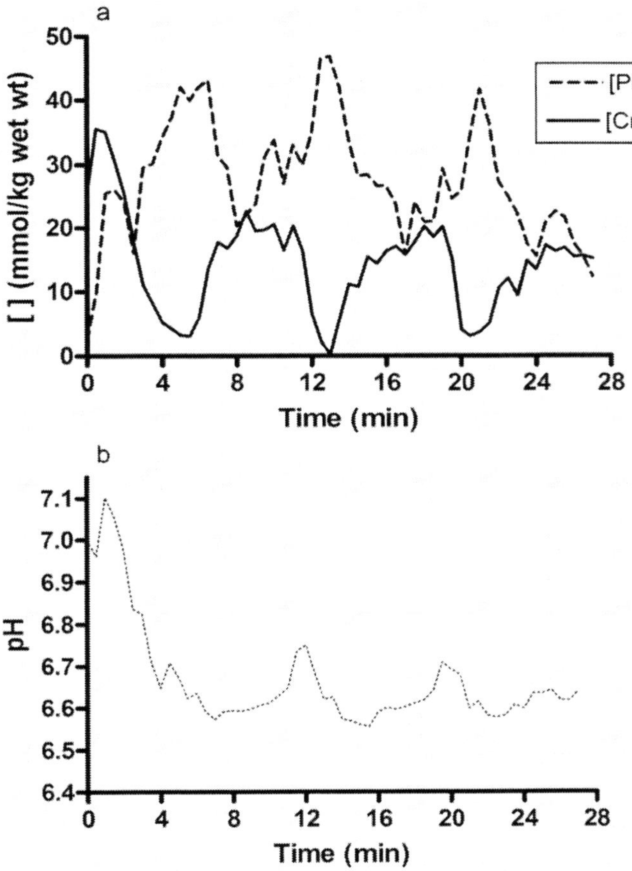

Figure 8. Data from a representative subject during repeated bouts of wrist flexion exercise (see text). a) The changes in creatine phosphate (CrP) and inorganic phosphate (Pi) during and in recovery from exercise. b) Changes in intramuscular pH revealing a sustained metabolic acidosis from bout 1 through bout 3.

Our most recent ^{31}P MRS investigation has produced very interesting data to compare to the in-vitro findings of Pedersen et al. [19]. As a reminder, this study revealed a benefit of intracellular acidosis to contractile force development in skinned muscle fibers from the rat due to a possible enhanced excitability of the t-tubule system. We designed a human subjects experiment where intense intermittent forearm wrist flexion exercise was performed. We measured the changes in muscle phosphate metabolites through exercise and recovery using ^{31}P MRS. Thus, we were able to assess the repeated ability of subjects to tax their phosphagen system through repeated intervals while accurately quantifying intramuscular pH. As pH recovery in muscle is a slow response, while CrP recovery is rapid, any delay in pH recovery, if intramuscular acidosis was influential to muscle fatigue, should detract from the subjects' capability to tax their phosphagen system in repeated intervals of exercise. Our data for a representative subject is presented in Figure 8. The subject completed 7 min of incremental exercise (1 kg increase/min @ 12 contractions/min), 5 min of recovery, then two additional bouts of intense exercise (2 min @ WLmax from exercise bout 1) to near failure separated by 5 min of recovery. The data are strikingly clear in showing the sustained condition of metabolic acidosis, yet the ability of the subject to continue to fully tax his phosphagen energy system while completing standard exercise. The data present no evidence intramuscular acidosis causing a detriment to in-vivo contractile function or cellular energy turnover.

The Importance of Proton Release from the Chemical Reactions of Non-Mitochondrial Energy Catabolism to Exercise-Induced Metabolic Acidosis

In the original manuscript where Peter Stewart introduced the theory of physico-chemical causes of acid-balance in blood and muscle, a key issue proposed was the sole dependence of the hydrogen ion activity of a solution on other, 'independent', variables such as the concentrations of positive and negatively charged elements and weak acids, and the partial pressure of CO_2 [53]. As such, Stewart indicated that tissues such as skeletal muscle did not alter body fluid acid-base balance by the production or release of protons during increasing metabolic demand. Consequently, the entire physico-chemical approach to acid-base chemistry has been interpreted to preclude recognition of a tissue contribution of protons to acid-base balance. For example, others have stated that "... the quantity of H^+ added or removed from a physiologic system is not relevant to the final pH, since [H+] is a 'dependent' variable ..." [54].

Clearly, one of the constraints of the Stewart approach is the treatment of H^+ activity (accumulation) as being solely dependent on other factors. This is an invalid assumption that today remains unsupported by any empirical data. Furthermore, to assume zero proton exchange from the sum of all reactions of cellular energy metabolism is in opposition to the exchange of protons, and other competing cations, based on computations from experimentally established dissociation constants for all known biological and non-biological organic molecules [55]. Clearly, the "Stewart" of "physico-chemical" approach to acid-base chemistry does not cause acidosis but demonstrates the potential for changes in ionic concentrations to alter cellular and blood proton balance. The important feature that is left to establish is the quantity of proton release, or what has been termed the "proton load", of intense muscle contraction.

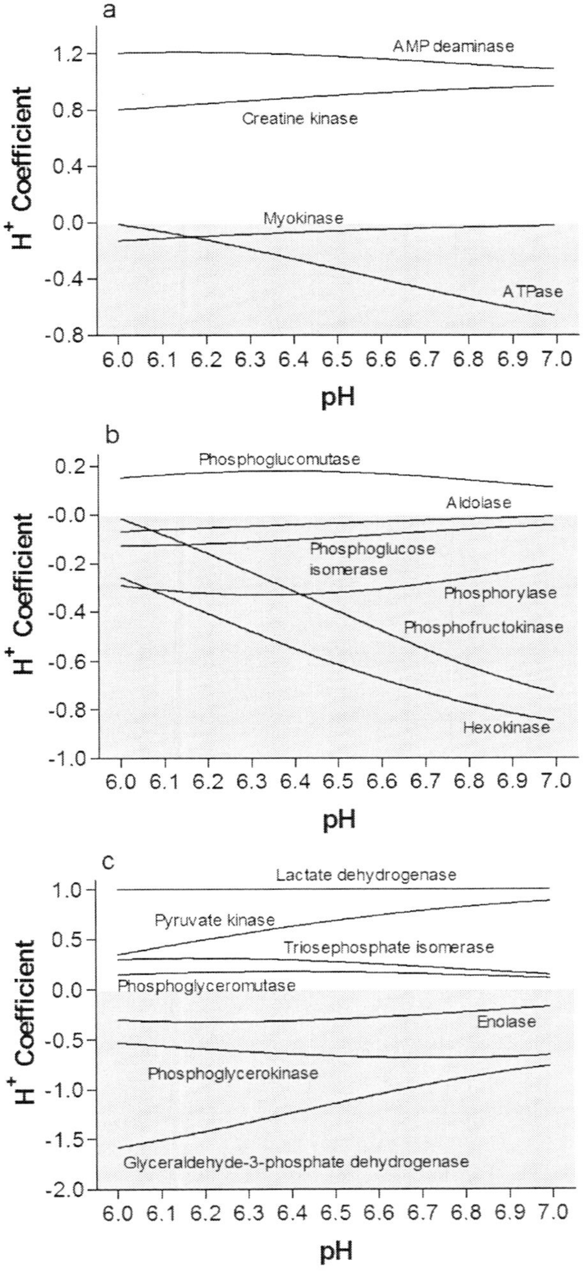

Figure 9. Computed data for proton coefficients from the reactions of non-mitochondrial energy catabolism in skeletal muscle. Negative coefficients represent H^+ release.

We believe an important contribution to understanding and quantifying the proton load of intense muscle contraction is to compute the proton coefficients of all metabolites and reactions of skeletal muscle non-mitochondrial energy metabolism (phosphagen and glycolytic energy systems). This work is based on acquiring known dissociation constants for multiple cations for specific metabolites from peer reviewed research [55]. We then computed the proportion of H^+, Na^+, K^+ and Mg^{++} dissociation for specific metabolites from pH 6.0 to 7.0 using an alpha equation as shown in Equation 2, which allowed us to develop proton coefficient curves across the physiological pH range for each metabolite.

$$\alpha_{-n} = \frac{[L^{n-}]}{L_{tot}} = \frac{1}{1 + K_H [H^+] + ... + K_{Hn} [H^+]^n + K_A [A^{a+}] + K_{AH} [A^{a+}][H^+] + ..}$$

Equation 2

(Note that for multiple cation binding, K_{AH} in equation 1 refers to K_H*K_{AH}, etc)

We then summed substrate (-'ve) and product (+'ve) H^+ coefficients for each reaction of the phosphagen and glycolytic systems to derive H^+ coefficient data for a given rate of product formation. For example, a H^+ coefficient of 1.0 would be 1.0 mmol/L H^+ release for 1 mmol/L product formation.

The results of this work were revealing of the specific reactions that contribute to, as well as oppose, proton release. In addition, the extent of net H^+ release possible from non-mitochondrial energy metabolism was shown to be remarkably high. Figure 9 presents the net H^+ coefficients for reactions of non-mitochondrial energy catabolism in skeletal muscle. Negative coefficients represent H^+ release. Interestingly, while most reactions are net H^+ releasing, the glyceraldehyde-3-phosphate dehydrogenase reaction is the most H^+ releasing reaction of glycolysis, with H^+ coefficients becoming more negative as pH decreases. Glycolysis sums to be net H^+ releasing when fueled from glycogen, with H^+ coefficients being -3.97 and -2.01 for pH 6 and 7, respectively.

When modeling muscle metabolism during 3 min of intense exercise to volitional exhaustion, net H^+ release amounts to approximately 80 mmol/kg wet wt. This H^+ load of intense muscle contraction is opposed by adjustment based on the ion constant of water, structural H^+ buffering, H^+ transport out of the muscle fiber, changes in strong ion concentrations, and additional chemical buffering by HCO_3^-. These data are revealing of the capacity of H^+ release by contracting skeletal muscle, and are more than double the previously accepted value based on the incorrect assumption of lactate production being stoichiometric to H^+ release.

METABOLIC ACIDOSIS AND FATIGUE: WHERE TO FROM HERE?

It is clear that the field of acid-base physiology is in a state of turmoil, with no accepted paradigm for explaining exercise-induced metabolic acidosis. The inability to understand the cause of metabolic acidosis, during exercise and even all other forms of acidosis, is a major detraction from the scientific advancement of basic, applied and clinical research and the application of these findings to professional practice. When viewed from the perspective of understanding fatigue and performance during exercise, current research interpretation clearly reveals the error of labeling acidosis and lactate production as fatigue inducing events. The notion that acidosis is the cause of contractile failure, and in particular that acidosis arose from the formation of a single molecule (lactate), is not a valid construct. The primary effects of acidosis appear to have a potential canceling effect. The slight loss in force production (as little as 10% based on in vitro studies) due to decreasing pH by impairment of myosin/actin binding as the H^+ competes with Ca^{++} at the troponin C site and through charge differential at the SR limiting Ca^{++} release may be offset by positive effects of a low pH on maintenance of action potential propagation through the t-system. Further research is needed to elucidate the effects of acidosis under in-vivo physiologic conditions to determine if even the slight loss in muscle force seen in vitro persists.

So what role does acidosis have to play in muscle fatigue? Our own ^{31}P MRS findings of sustained near maximal ATP turnover from the phosphagen system during repeated intense exercise intervals despite continued metabolic acidosis (Figure 8), clearly reveals a disconnect between acidosis and fatigue. Interestingly, one area of influence of acidosis to fatigue may be outside of the muscle cell. There is evidence that the H^+ directly affects group IV afferents that are chemically sensitive [56]. Increased afferent discharge from neurons that provide nociception have been shown to inhibit the motor neuron pool which could decrease alpha motor neuron firing thus reducing force production [57-61]. Hodges [59] demonstrated that experimentally induced pain in the triceps surae complex reduced motor unit firing rates by as much as 12%. Additionally, the synergistic muscles that would contribute to continued force production also showed decreased motor neuron firing rates.

During muscle fatigue the discharge of these small-diameter muscle afferents (groups III and IV) increases according to the temperature, chemical and the mechanical environment of their free nerve endings, which are all altered during intense exercise and thus can contribute to fatigue [62]. Lastly, further input from group IV afferents that are stimulated repeatedly by increasing $[H^+]$ may have an effect on central processing by the cortex, particularly the enkephalinergic, dopaminergic and serotonergic systems, which appear to control motivation, pain and vigilance [62]. Processing in these regions of the brain could lead to increased pain perception and thus contribute to the bottom of the fatigue curve, particularly the decision to end exercise.

References

[1] Robergs R, Ghiasvand F, Parker D. Biochemistry of exercise-induced metabolic acidosis. *Am J Physiol Regul Integr Comp Physiol*, 2004, 287, R502.

[2] Arnold D, Matthews P, Radda G. Metabolic recovery after exercise and the assessment of mitochondrial function in vivo in human skeletal muscle by means of 31P NMR. *Magn Reson Med*, 1984, 1, 307-15.

[3] Siegler JC, Bell-Wilson J, Mermier C, Faria E, Robergs RA. Active and passive recovery and acid-base kinetics following multiple bouts of intense exercise to exhaustion. *Int J Sport Nutr Exerc Metab*, 2006, 16, 92-107.

[4] Robergs R, Hutchinson K, Hendee S, Madden S, Siegler J. Influence of pre-exercise acidosis and alkalosis on the kinetics of acid-base recovery following intense exercise. *Int J Sport Nutr Exerc Metab*, 2005, 15, 59.

[5] Juel C. Lactate-proton cotransport in skeletal muscle. *Physiol Rev*, 1997, 77, 321.

[6] Juel C. Training-induced changes in membrane transport proteins of human skeletal muscle. *Eur J Appl Physiol*, 2006, 96, 627-35.

[7] Juel C. Regulation of pH in human skeletal muscle: adaptations to physical activity. *Acta Physiol*, 2008, 193, 17-24.

[8] Juel C, Klarskov C, Nielsen J, Krustrup P, Mohr M, Bangsbo J. Effect of high-intensity intermittent training on lactate and H+ release from human skeletal muscle. *Am J Physiol Endocrinol Metab*, 2004, 286, E245.

[9] Messonnier L, Kristensen M, Juel C, Denis C. Importance of pH regulation and lactate/H+ transport capacity for work production during supramaximal exercise in humans. *J Appl Physiol*, 2007, 102, 1936.

[10] Cairns S. Lactic acid and exercise performance: culprit or friend? *Sports Med*, 2006, 36, 279-91.

[11] Fitts R. Cellular mechanisms of muscle fatigue. *Physiol Rev*, 1994, 74, 49.

[12] Gladden L. 200th anniversary of lactate research in muscle. *Exerc Sport Sci Rev*, 2008, 36, 109.

[13] Sahlin K. Intracellular pH and energy metabolism in skeletal muscle of man. With special reference to exercise. *Acta Physiol Scand Suppl*, 1978, 455, 1.

[14] Sahlin K, Harris R, Hultman E. Creatine kinase equilibrium and lactate content compared with muscle pH in tissue samples obtained after isometric exercise. *Biochem J*, 1975, 152, 173.

[15] Sahlin K, Harris R, Nylind B, Hultman E. Lactate content and pH in muscle samples obtained after dynamic exercise. *Pflugers Arch*, 1976, 367, 143-9.

[16] Hermansen L, Osnes J. Blood and muscle pH after maximal exercise in man. *J Appl Physiol*, 1972, 32, 304.

[17] Adams R, Welch H. Oxygen uptake, acid-base status, and performance with varied inspired oxygen fractions. *J Appl Physiol*, 1980, 49, 863.

[18] Hogan M, Richardson R, Haseler L. Human muscle performance and PCr hydrolysis with varied inspired oxygen fractions: a 31P-MRS study. *J Appl Physiol*, 1999, 86, 1367.

[19] Pedersen T, Nielsen O, Lamb G, Stephenson D. Intracellular acidosis enhances the excitability of working muscle. *Sci*, 2004, 305, 1144.

[20] Sostaric S. Alkalosis increases muscle K+ release, but lowers plasma [K+] and delays fatigue during dynamic forearm exercise. *J Physiol*, 2006, 570, 185.

[21] Street D, Nielsen J, Bangsbo J, Juel C. Metabolic alkalosis reduces exercise-induced acidosis and potassium accumulation in human skeletal muscle interstitium. *J Physiol*, 2005, 566, 481.

[22] Hultman E, Sahlin K. Acid-base balance during exercise. *Exerc Sport Sci Rev*, 1980, 8, 41.

[23] Brooks G, Dubouchaud H, Brown M, Sicurello J, Butz C. Role of mitochondrial lactate dehydrogenase and lactate oxidation in the intracellular lactate shuttle. *Proc Natl Acad Sci U S A*, 1999, 96, 1129.

[24] Hashimoto T, Hussien R, Brooks G. Colocalization of MCT1, CD147, and LDH in mitochondrial inner membrane of L6 muscle cells: evidence of a mitochondrial lactate oxidation complex. *Am J Physiol Endocrinol Metab*, 2006, 290, E1237.

[25] Ball D, Maughan R. The effect of sodium citrate ingestion on the metabolic response to intense exercise following diet manipulation in man. *Exp Physiol*, 1997, 82, 1041.

[26] Kowalchuk J, Maltais S, Yamaji K, Hughson R. The effect of citrate loading on exercise performance, acid-base balance and metabolism. *Eur J Appl Physiol Occup Physiol*, 1989, 58, 858-64.

[27] Parry-Billings M, MacLaren D. The effect of sodium bicarbonate and sodium citrate ingestion on anaerobic power during intermittent exercise. *Eur J Appl Physiol Occup Physiol*, 1986, 55, 524-9.

[28] Dennig H, Talbott J, Edwards H, Dill D. Effect of acidosis and alkalosis upon capacity for work. *J Clin Invest*, 1931, 9, 601.

[29] Goldfinch J, McNaughton L, Davies P. Bicarbonate ingestion and its effects upon 400-m racing time. *Eur J Appl Physiol Occup Physiol*, 1988, 57, 45-8.

[30] Mc Naughton L, Cedaro R. Sodium citrate ingestion and its effects on maximal anaerobic exercise of different durations. *Eur J Appl Physiol Occup Physiol*, 1992, 64, 36-41.

[31] Raymer G, Marsh G, Kowalchuk J, Thompson R. Metabolic effects of induced alkalosis during progressive forearm exercise to fatigue. *J Appl Physiol*, 2004, 96, 2050.

[32] Requena B, Zabala M, Padial P, Feriche B. Sodium Bicarbonate and Sodium Citrate: Ergogenic AIDS? *J Strength Cond Res*, 2005, 19, 213.

[33] Wilkes D, Gledhill N, Smyth R. Effect of acute induced metabolic alkalosis on 800-m racing time. *Med Sci Sports Exerc*, 1983, 15, 277.

[34] Spriet L, Soderlund K, Bergstrom M, Hultman E. Skeletal muscle glycogenolysis, glycolysis, and pH during electrical stimulation in men. *J Appl Physiol*, 1987, 62, 616.

[35] Sullivan M, Saltin B, Negro-Vilar R, Duscha B, Charles H. Skeletal muscle pH assessed by biochemical and 31P-MRS methods during exercise and recovery in men. *J Appl Physiol*, 1994, 77, 2194.

[36] Cooke R, Pate E. The effects of ADP and phosphate on the contraction of muscle fibers. *BpJ*, 1985, 48, 789-98.

[37] Donaldsen S, Hermansen K. Differential, direct effect of H+ on Ca2+-activated force of skinned fibers from soleus, cardiac and adductor magnus muscles of rabbit. *Pflugers Arch*, 1978, 376, 55-65.

[38] Edman K, Mattiazzi A. Effects of fatigue and altered pH on isometric force and velocity of shortening at zero load in frog muscle fibres. *J Muscle Res Cell Motil*, 1981, 2, 321-34.

[39] Fabiato A, Fabiato F. Effects of pH on the myofilaments and the sarcoplasmic reticulum of skinned cells from cardiace and skeletal muscles. *J Physiol*, 1978, 276, 233.

[40] Metzger J, Fitts R. Role of intracellular pH in muscle fatigue. *J Appl Physiol*, 1987, 62, 1392.

[41] Trivedi B, Danforth W. Effect of pH on the kinetics of frog muscle phosphofructokinase. *J Biol Chem*, 1966, 241, 4110.

[42] Spriet L. ATP utilization and provision in fast-twitch skeletal muscle during tetanic contractions. *Am J Physiol Endocrinol Metab*, 1989, 257, E595.

[43] Bangsbo J, Graham T, Johansen L, Strange S, Christensen C, Saltin B. Elevated muscle acidity and energy production during exhaustive exercise in humans. *Am J Physiol Regul Integr Comp Physiol*, 1992, 263, 891.

[44] Bangsbo J, Johansen L, Graham T, Saltin B. Lactate and H+ effluxes from human skeletal muscles during intense, dynamic exercise. *J Physiol*, 1993, 462, 115.

[45] Bangsbo J, Madsen K, Kiens B, Richter E. Effect of muscle acidity on muscle metabolism and fatigue during intense exercise in man. *J Physiol*, 1996, 495, 587.

[46] Pate E, Bhimani M, Franks-Skiba K, Cooke R. Reduced effect of pH on skinned rabbit psoas muscle mechanics at high temperatures: implications for fatigue. *J Physiol*, 1995, 486, 689.

[47] Westerblad H, Bruton J, Lännergren J. The effect of intracellular pH on contractile function of intact, single fibres of mouse muscle declines with increasing temperature. *J Physiol*, 1997, 500, 193.

[48] Knuth ST, Dave H, Peters JR, Fitts RH. Low cell pH depresses peak power in rat skeletal muscle fibres at both 30 degrees C and 15 degrees C: implications for muscle fatigue. *J Physiol*, 2006, 575, 887-99.

[49] Fitts R. The cross-bridge cycle and skeletal muscle fatigue. *J Appl Physiol*, 2008, 104, 551.

[50] Nielsen O, de Paoli F, Overgaard K. Protective effects of lactic acid on force production in rat skeletal muscle. *J Physiol*, 2001, 536, 161.

[51] Kemp G, Meyerspeer M, Moser E. Absolute quantification of phosphorus metabolite concentrations in human muscle in vivo by 31P MRS: a quantitative review. *NMR Biomed*, 2007, 20, 555-65.

[52] Smith SA, Montain SJ, Zientara GP, Fielding RA. Use of phosphocreatine kinetics to determine the influence of creatine on muscle mitochondrial respiration: an in vivo 31P-MRS study of oral creatine ingestion. *J Appl Physiol*, 2004, 96, 2288-92.

[53] Stewart P. Modern quantitative acid-base chemistry. *Can J Physiol Pharmacol*, 1983, 61, 1444-61.

[54] Corey H. Stewart and beyond: new models of acid-base balance. *Kidney Int*, 2003, 64, 777-87.

[55] National Institute of Standards and Technology. NIST critically selected stability constants of metal complexes database. NIST standard reference database. Gaithersburg, Maryland: 1994.

[56] Hoheisel U, Reinöhl J, Unger T, Mense S. Acidic pH and capsaicin activate mechanosensitive group IV muscle receptors in the rat. *Pain*, 2004, 110, 149-57.

[57] Birznieks I, Burton A, Macefield V. The effects of experimental muscle and skin pain on the static stretch sensitivity of human muscle spindles in relaxed leg muscles. *J Physiol*, 2008, 586, 2713.

[58] Graven-Nielsen T, Lund H, Arendt-Nielsen L, Danneskiold-Samsøe B, Bliddal H. Inhibition of maximal voluntary contraction force by experimental muscle pain: a centrally mediated mechanism. *Muscle Nerve*, 2002, 26, 708-12.

[59] Hodges P, Ervilha U, Graven-Nielsen T. Changes in motor unit firing rate in synergist muscles cannot explain the maintenance of force during constant force painful contractions. *J Pain*, 2008, 9, 1169-74.

[60] Kniffki K, Schomburg E, Steffens H. Synaptic effects from chemically activated fine muscle afferents upon [alpha]-motoneurones in decerebrate and spinal cats. *Brain Res*, 1981, 206, 361-70.
[61] Rossi A, Mazzocchio R, Decchi B. Effect of chemically activated fine muscle afferents on spinal recurrent inhibition in humans. *Clin Neurophysiol*, 2003, 114, 279-87.
[62] Gandevia SC. Neural control in human muscle fatigue: changes in muscle afferents, moto neurones and moto cortical drive. *Acta Physiol Scand*, 1998, 162, 275-83.

In: Regulation of Fatigue in Exercise
Editor: Frank E. Marino
ISBN 978-1-61209-334-5

Chapter 4

CENTRAL MECHANISMS LIMITING MUSCLE PERFORMANCE IN FATIGUE

***Janet L. Taylor**, *Simon C. Gandevia*,**
Neuroscience Research Australia and the University of New South Wales
Barker St, Randwick, NSW 2031, Australia

ABSTRACT

During exercise, muscle fatigue leads to a loss of maximal voluntary force or power. Processes in the muscle contribute to fatigue, but there is also a contribution from processes in the nervous system. This is known as central fatigue. Central fatigue is demonstrated when twitch interpolation shows a progressive failure of voluntary activation. That is, the motoneurones fire too slowly to generate maximal possible muscle force despite maximal voluntary effort. During single limb exercise, factors that influence the development of central fatigue are primarily repetitive activation of neurones in the motor pathway and changes in inputs to these neurones from other motor areas or from sensory feedback. At a spinal level, changes in the intrinsic properties of motoneurones make them harder to drive, and descending drive from the motor cortex becomes less effective. Supraspinal fatigue can be identified using transcranial magnetic stimulation, which shows that extra output from the motor cortex is available but remains untapped by voluntary effort. The mechanism for this is unknown but feedback from fatigue-sensitive small-diameter muscle afferents may be important. During whole-body exercise, the addition of systemic changes is likely to cause further impairment of the performance of the motor pathway.

* Email: j.taylor@neura.edu.au; Phone +61 2 9399 1116

Introduction

Exercise is sustained or repetitive activation of one or more muscle groups. In people, voluntary muscle contractions are driven primarily from the motor cortex through corticospinal neurones which act at a spinal level to activate motoneurones directly and indirectly. Each motoneurone innervates a group of muscle fibres and their contraction produces force and/or movement. During exercise, changes occur at most levels in this chain. Some of the changes contribute to an impairment of the force produced by the muscle. That is, they contribute to muscle fatigue, which can be defined as any exercise-induced reduction in the ability of a muscle or muscle group to generate force or power [1, 2].

It is useful to consider three ways that exercise can alter the motor pathway. First, neurones and muscle fibres fire repeatedly and there are intrinsic changes in their behaviour that are related to this repetitive activation [e.g. 3, 4]. Second, the firing of neurones and muscle fibres depends on their input and this input can change with fatigue. Muscle fibres only have input from the motoneurones that innervate them, but the motoneurones receive input from sensory receptors, as well as descending drive. Motor cortical cells receive inputs from multiple cortical and subcortical areas including sensory feedback from the periphery. In particular, sensory receptors in muscle are activated by muscle contraction and affected by fatigue, and these feed back to the neurones in the motor pathway at both a spinal and a cortical level. Third, there are systemic effects associated with whole-body exercise that may influence motor output especially under particular conditions, such as hyperthermia, decreased glucose availability, decreased oxygen availability, blood flow limitations, and other metabolic changes. It is important to note that systemic effects may influence muscle fibres or the neurones in the motor pathway directly, or indirectly via activation of afferents. Systemic effects will not be addressed here as this chapter is concerned primarily with the contribution of the nervous system to fatigue in single limb exercise.

While it is clear that processes related to excitation and contraction of the muscle contribute greatly to the impairment of maximal force output with fatigue [e.g. 5], processes in the nervous system also contribute. This contribution is known as central fatigue and, for practical reasons, is considered to encompass processes above the level of the terminal branches of the motor axons, whereas peripheral fatigue includes processes in the terminal branches, neuromuscular junction and muscle fibres (see Figure 1)[6, 7]. Central fatigue can be defined as a progressive reduction in the voluntary activation of muscle during exercise [2]. That is, a decline in the ability of the nervous system to drive the muscle maximally. In addition, supraspinal fatigue can be identified as a subclass of central fatigue. It can be defined as fatigue produced by failure to generate output from the motor cortex [2].

Measurement of Voluntary Activation

Motor Nerve Stimulation

Voluntary activation can be measured using the technique of twitch interpolation [6, 7]. Here, maximal stimulation of the motor nerve to a muscle is carried out during a maximal voluntary contraction (MVC). If an increment in force is evoked despite the subject's maximal effort then voluntary activation is less than 100%. Some motor units are either not recruited or are not firing fast enough to form fused contractions. To quantify the level of voluntary activation, the increment in force (superimposed twitch) is compared to the twitch of the muscle at rest. As ongoing or previous activity can potentiate the force evoked from a muscle, the superimposed twitch is potentiated and so should be compared to a potentiated resting twitch elicited shortly after a maximal effort. Voluntary activation is expressed as a percentage and can be calculated using the formula, voluntary activation = (1- superimposed twitch/resting twitch) X 100 [6, 8, 9]. Voluntary activation is commonly high in isometric MVCs but is rarely 100% [2, 8]. It is frequently measured with motor nerve stimulation in the knee extensors (85-95%), elbow flexors (>95%), ankle dorsiflexors (95-100%) and plantarflexors (>95%), and the diaphragm. It has also been measured in elbow extensors, intrinsic hand muscles, abdominal muscles, and masseter [2, 10].

When measuring voluntary activation during a fatiguing protocol, two additional points should be kept in mind. First, the repeated activation of motoneurones by voluntary activity changes the threshold of their axons for electrical stimulation irrespective of any change in their response to voluntary drive. After a 1-min MVC, there is a 30% increase in threshold, so that unless the stimulus is sufficiently supramaximal initially, it will no longer activate all of the muscle [11]. Second, the contractile response of the muscle to a single action potential is more affected by fatigue than the response to repetitive activation [12, 13]. Thus, the resting twitch to a single stimulus may decrease disproportionately compared to the superimposed twitch and overemphasise a failure of voluntary activation. The use of a pair of stimuli at high frequency (100 Hz) can ameliorate this problem.

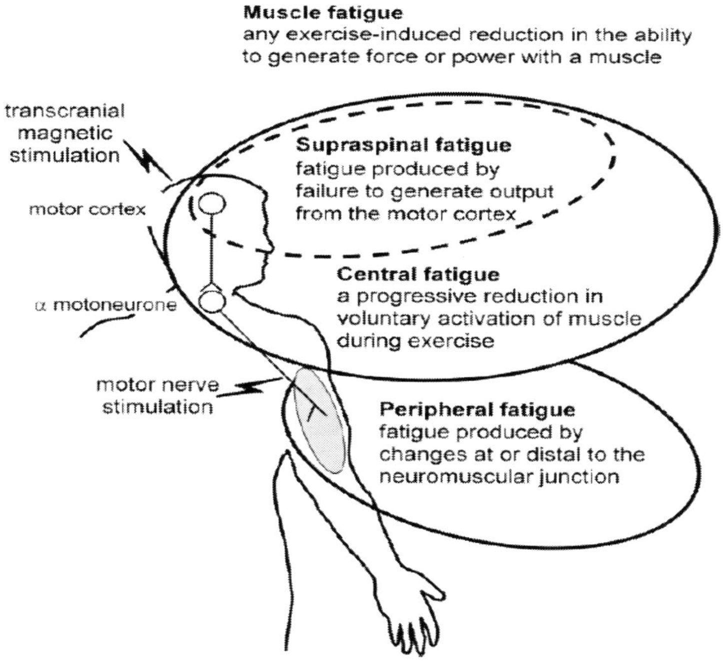

Figure 1. Definitions of muscle fatigue, peripheral fatigue, central fatigue and supraspinal fatigue. Peripheral and central fatigue can be identified by stimulation of the motor nerve. Supraspinal fatigue is a component of central fatigue. It can be identified by transcranial stimulation over the motor cortex.

Motor Cortex Stimulation

Voluntary activation can also be measured using transcranial magnetic stimulation over the motor cortex rather than stimulation of the motor nerve [14-18]. Again the stimulus is delivered during a MVC and if an increment in force is evoked, then voluntary activation is less than 100%. However, a failure of voluntary activation measured with cortical stimulation has different implications than that measured with motor nerve stimulation. It indicates that extra output could be evoked from the motor cortex, motoneurones and muscle despite maximal voluntary effort. It implies that motor cortical output was not maximal and was not sufficient to drive the motoneurones maximally and that motoneurone firing was not maximal and was not sufficient to drive the muscle fibres maximally. Voluntary activation measured with motor cortical stimulation can be quantified but it is not appropriate to compare the superimposed twitch to the twitch evoked by stimulation with the muscle at rest. Excitability at both cortical and spinal levels increases with voluntary contraction so that the effective input to the muscle from the same cortical stimulus is much less during rest than during contraction. To circumvent this problem, an estimated resting twitch can be calculated from the relationship between the superimposed twitch and voluntary force. For the elbow flexor muscles, this relationship is linear for voluntary contractions of above 50% maximal and the amplitude of the estimated resting twitch is calculated by extrapolation to the axis (zero voluntary force) [17]. The estimated resting twitch can then be used in the formula, Voluntary activation = (1-superimposed twitch/estimated resting twitch) X 100. For the elbow flexors, voluntary activation measured with cortical stimulation is reported as 90-95%. The technique has also been used for the wrist flexors and knee extensors [15, 16]. In addition, cortical stimulation has been used to evoke superimposed twitches from adductor pollicis and the elbow extensors [19, 20].

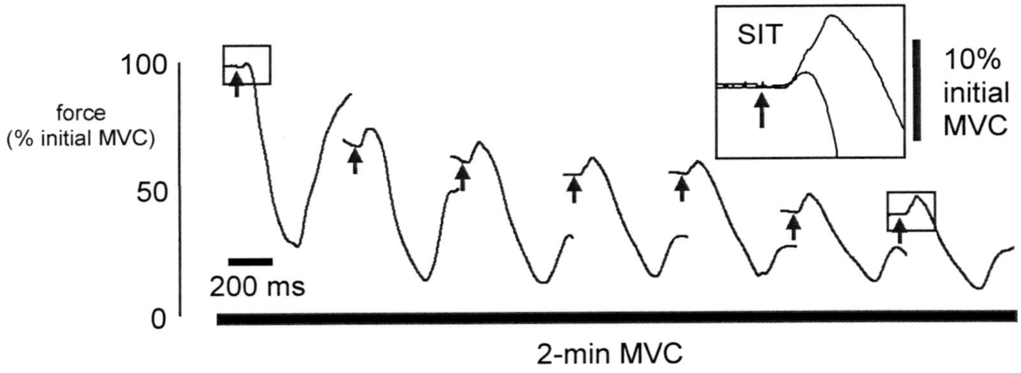

Figure 2. Traces of elbow flexion force recorded at intervals during a sustained maximal voluntary contraction (MVC) of the elbow flexor muscles. Each trace is around the time of transcranial magnetic stimulation over the motor cortex (black arrows). The progressive fall in force before the stimuli shows the development of fatigue during the sustained MVC. After each stimulus, there is a small increment in force (superimposed twitch, SIT). The SIT is small at the start of the fatiguing contraction and larger later in the contraction. This indicates supraspinal fatigue. SITs from the first and final traces are shown enlarged in the inset. The fall in force after each SIT corresponds to the silent period, in which voluntary EMG is suppressed.

Problems with the use of cortical stimulation to measure voluntary activation include the difficulty in localising stimulation to one muscle or muscle group. Stimulation of the antagonist muscle in addition to the agonist reduces the size of the superimposed twitch [17]. Submaximal stimulation of the motoneurone pool and muscle can also be a problem. It produces small superimposed twitches in the lower force contractions and results in a small estimated resting twitch.

EVIDENCE FOR CENTRAL FATIGUE

During fatiguing exercise, there is a decline in the ability of the nervous system to activate muscles maximally. This decline represents central fatigue and is demonstrated by a fall in voluntary activation (or an increase in the size of the superimposed twitch). It can be demonstrated during different kinds of exercise and for different muscles including the knee extensors, ankle plantar and dorsiflexors, elbow flexors, diaphragm and hand muscles [2].

One of the most straightforward paradigms for causing muscle fatigue is the maintenance of an isometric maximal voluntary effort of a single muscle group. Here, within a few seconds, fatigue is apparent as a fall in force. At the same time a progressive increase in the superimposed twitch evoked by motor nerve stimulation shows that central fatigue develops [14, 21-24]. At the end of a 1.5-3 min MVC, voluntary activation is reported to fall by 10-15% [14, 22]. Demonstration of central fatigue with motor nerve stimulation implies that motoneuronal drive to the muscle has become worse at producing fused contractions of all the motor units, but it gives no indication of the mechanism for inadequate drive to the muscle. If motor cortical stimulation is delivered during a sustained MVC, then the superimposed twitches which it evokes also grow progressively (Figure 2) [14, 25, 26]. This growth indicates that voluntary drive from the motor cortex has become worse at driving the motoneurones. Although additional motor cortical output can be accessed by the stimulus, it is not employed voluntarily despite the subject's maximal voluntary effort. Thus, the increase in the superimposed twitch to motor cortex stimulation suggests that some of central fatigue is due to mechanisms at a supraspinal level and is a marker of supraspinal fatigue [27]. Theoretically, comparison of voluntary activation measured with motor nerve stimulation and motor cortical stimulation should quantify the supraspinal contribution to central fatigue. However, in practice, non-linearities in the relationship between voluntary force and voluntary activation measured with motor nerve stimulation mean that this is not possible [17]. Central and supraspinal fatigue are seen not only during sustained isometric maximal efforts but also during intermittent isometric and dynamic maximal efforts [28-32].

Although it is less obvious than during maximal contractions, fatigue also develops during submaximal exercise. If a contraction to a target force is maintained, the active muscle fibres gradually fatigue and EMG increases progressively as more motor units are recruited to compensate [9, 33, 34]. If brief MVCs are performed occasionally through the submaximal exercise, a fall in maximal voluntary force is seen [9, 34-37]. As central and supraspinal fatigue are demonstrated by the failure of the nervous system to activate the muscle maximally, measurement of voluntary activation during submaximal forces is not helpful in identifying central fatigue [38]. However, motor nerve and motor cortical stimulation delivered during brief MVCs performed during a sustained submaximal contraction show that central and supraspinal fatigue do develop [36, 37]. This occurs during contractions as weak as 5% maximum if they are maintained for long enough [35]. Indeed, ~two-thirds of the loss of maximal force during a 5% contraction held for >1 hour was explained by supraspinal fatigue, whereas supraspinal fatigue accounts for ~one quarter of fatigue during a 2-min MVC [27, 35].

Whole-body exercise such as cycling or running can also produce central fatigue in the muscles that are used in the exercise [39]. For example, following running or cycling, stimulation of the femoral nerve shows an increase in the superimposed twitch during maximal isometric knee extension [40, 41]. Furthermore, in a recent study, cortical stimulation delivered during isometric MVCs after cycling showed a supraspinal contribution to central fatigue [25]. Surprisingly, this failure of cortical drive to the knee extensors had not recovered by 45 minutes after the end of exercise and was exacerbated during sustained contractions.

Taken together, it seems that central fatigue develops along with peripheral fatigue during most exercise and that, whenever it has been tested, there is a supraspinal component to the central fatigue. The contribution of central fatigue varies with the kind of exercise but under some conditions it can be as important, or more important, than peripheral mechanisms for loss of force [38]. The mechanisms of central fatigue are not clear but are likely to include processes at a spinal and cortical level, and they ultimately result in motoneurone firing that is insufficient to activate muscles to generate their maximal available force output.

MOTONEURONES DURING FATIGUE

During a sustained maximal voluntary contraction, the muscle fibre relaxation rates slow [42-44]. Thus, fused contractions of the fibres can be maintained despite some decrease in motor unit firing rates. However, the presence of an increasing superimposed twitch indicates that motoneurone firing slows too much to maintain full activation of the muscle and so contributes to fatigue. Motoneurone firing depends on the properties of the motoneurones and on their synaptic input from afferents and descending drive. During fatiguing exercise, a reduction in firing rates could result from a change in motoneurone properties that make the motoneurones less responsive to input, or an increase in inhibitory input, or a decrease in excitatory drive. Some inputs to motoneurones come from muscle afferents which are likely to change during contraction and fatigue. These afferents include those from the muscle spindles (groups Ia and II), from Golgi tendon organs (Ib) and the small-diameter myelinated and unmyelinated afferents (groups III and IV). Muscle spindle afferents fire during voluntary contractions and a reduction in their firing and an increase in presynaptic inhibition during sustained contractions may reduce excitation to the motoneurones of the fatigued muscle and could contribute to decreased firing rates [45-47]. Tendon organ inhibition to the contracting muscle is reduced during sustained voluntary contractions so that it is unlikely to reduce motoneurone firing [48-50]. The influence of small-diameter afferents is addressed in a subsequent section.

Some insight into motoneurone behaviour during fatigue in humans can be gained from examining responses to stimulation of the corticospinal tract. An electrical pulse passed between the mastoid processes activates corticospinal axons at the cervicomedullary junction to evoke a single descending volley [51, 52]. This in turn activates motoneurones and produces a response which can be measured in the electromyogram (EMG). During a sustained MVC, these responses (cervicomedullary motor evoked potentials, CMEPs) decrease in size compared to the maximal compound muscle action potential (Mmax) evoked by peripheral nerve stimulation (Figure 3A,C)[53, 54]. Thus, motoneurone excitability decreases. The decrease in CMEP size during a strong contraction is not compatible with a decrease in excitatory drive to the motoneurones but indicates that the motoneurones have become harder to drive either through inhibition or through a change in their intrinsic properties [55]. The behaviour of individual motor units during sustained submaximal contractions suggests that changes in the intrinsic properties of motor units occur with repetitive activation. Motoneurones that are continuously activated become less responsive to synaptic input [56, 57]. They require more voluntary drive to maintain their firing rates and can even cease firing [58]. As this behaviour is specific to motoneurones which have been firing for some time, it is unlikely to be due to a change in input to the motoneurone pool. Such changes should also affect newly recruited motoneurones. Overall, the slowing of motoneurone firing cannot be due solely to a decrease in excitatory drive and a contribution from altered intrinsic properties of the motoneurones due to their repetitive activation is likely.

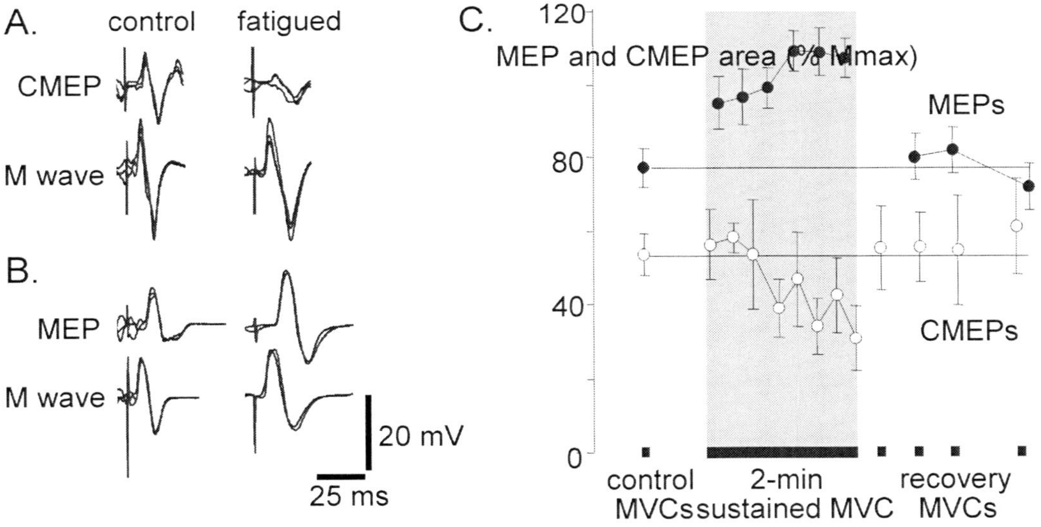

Figure 3. Changes in motor evoked potentials (MEPs) and cervicomedullary motor evoked potentials (CMEPs) during a sustained maximal voluntary contraction (MVC). A. Overlaid traces of CMEPs and maximal M waves (evoked through brachial plexus stimulation) recorded from biceps brachii in one subject during brief MVCs (control) and near the end of a 2-min MVC (fatigued). B. Overlaid traces of MEPs and maximal M waves recorded from biceps brachii in one subject during brief MVCs (control) and near the end of a 2-min MVC (fatigued). C. The area of MEPs and CMEPs during a 2-min MVC and during brief MVCs before and after the sustained contraction. Each potential in each subject was normalised to the maximal M wave (Mmax) recorded at close to the same time. MEPs and CMEPs were recorded in two separate studies.

Motor Cortex during Fatigue

Motor cortical excitability can be examined during voluntary contractions using transcranial magnetic stimulation (TMS). Here, a pulsed magnetic field induces an electrical current in the cortex and activates neurones. When delivered over the primary motor cortex TMS evokes a short-latency excitatory response in the EMG (motor evoked potential, MEP). Pyramidal tract neurones are activated directly by stimulation of their axons or indirectly through synapses by stimulation of cortico-cortical neurones [59, 60]. The indirect stimulation means that the size of responses evoked in the descending axons is influenced by the excitability of neurones in the cortex. Because responses are recorded in the EMG, they are also influenced by the excitability of the motoneurones. During voluntary contractions, the MEP is followed by a lengthy period of EMG silence. The latter part of this silent period is thought to be due to intracortical inhibition via $GABA_B$ receptors so that the duration of the silent period represents the actions of inhibitory interneurones in the cortex [e.g. 61, 62].

During a sustained MVC, supraspinal fatigue increases. That is, motor cortical output becomes less able to drive the muscle fully [14, 26]. EMG responses to cortical stimulation also change [63]. The MEP grows in size (Figure 3 B, C). As the decrease in CMEP at the same time shows a reduction in the excitability of the motoneurones, the increase in the MEP suggests that the motor cortex becomes more excitable [53, 64]. Similarly, fMRI studies show that the BOLD signal at first increases during a sustained maximal effort although then it decreases [65]. However, while the MEP grows, the silent period also lengthens and this suggests an increase in inhibition in the cortex [64]. These paradoxical changes make it difficult to understand what cortical changes underlie the increase in supraspinal fatigue. Furthermore, under some circumstances supraspinal fatigue can be dissociated from the changes in the MEP and silent period so that neither is critical for the development of supraspinal fatigue [14, 64].

Paired pulse TMS has also been used to investigate intracortical inhibition with fatigue. In these paradigms, a conditioning TMS pulse is used to alter the MEP evoked by a subsequent stimulus. Short-interval intracortical inhibition (SICI) is thought to be mediated by $GABA_A$ receptors and long-interval intracortical inhibition (LICI) by $GABA_B$ receptors, like the silent period. Both SICI and LICI have been tested with the muscle at rest during and after fatiguing exercise which consisted of intermittent contractions, and both decreased progressively with fatigue [66-68]. This contrasts with the increase in the silent period which occurs when the muscle is contracting. When LICI is tested during a sustained MVC, it increases dramatically but this appears to be through spinal rather than cortical mechanisms [69]. Thus, it seems that inhibition in the motor cortex may not contribute to supraspinal fatigue.

Groups III and IV Muscle Afferents

Afferent input from the limbs alters the excitability of neurones in the motor pathway at a spinal and cortical level. While cutaneous input does influence the motor pathway, the input that is most likely to change during fatiguing exercise is from the muscles. In particular, small-diameter (groups III and IV) muscle afferents are thought to have a role during fatigue as some of them are chemically sensitive and increase their firing with the accumulation of metabolites, while others are mechanically sensitive and fire with contractions [70-74]. The firing of both mechanically and chemically sensitive afferents is enhanced by ischemia. It is group III and IV muscle afferents that transduce muscle pain and contribute to the sensations of muscle fatigue with exercise.

The role of small-diameter muscle afferents in fatigue appears to be complex. It has been postulated that they provide reflex inhibition to motoneurones but this is not true for all muscle groups [54]. When muscle is held ischaemic at the end of a fatiguing contraction by blocking blood flow to the limb, metabolites are held within the muscle and its recovery is prevented. Under these conditions, a period of relaxation allows the motor cortex and motoneurones to recover from any effects of repetitive activation but the group III and IV afferents continue to fire [14, 75, 76]. With fatigue of quadriceps, maintained ischemia keeps motor unit firing rates slow, and for the ankle plantar flexors, H-reflexes are decreased [76, 77]. However, these changes could result from presynaptic inhibition of Ia inputs by group III and IV afferents [47, 78]. When motoneurone pools supplying arm muscles are tested with CMEPs during brief MVCs, responses in triceps brachii are inhibited, whereas those in biceps brachii are not [54]. Indeed, CMEPs in biceps are even facilitated with fatigue of the elbow extensor muscles, whereas those in triceps are inhibited with fatigue of the antagonist elbow flexor muscles. Thus, at the spinal cord, group III and IV muscle afferent firing maintained by ischemia after a fatiguing contraction inhibits some motoneurone pools but can excite others. It cannot account for the decrease in the response to corticospinal tract stimulation observed in biceps brachii during a sustained MVC, but it could contribute to motoneurone slowing and central fatigue in other muscle groups [53, 54].

Small-diameter muscle afferents can also have a supraspinal influence on fatigue. When TMS is carried out at rest during ischemia after a fatiguing effort, MEPs are unaffected [79]. Similarly, during brief MVCs during maintained ischemia, the recovery of MEPs and the silent period is unaffected [14]. However, the superimposed twitch evoked from the elbow flexors remains large. This supraspinal fatigue only recovers when blood flow to the arm is allowed to resume. Thus, despite no apparent direct effect on the primary motor cortex, small-diameter afferents contribute to supraspinal fatigue. During cycling, a reduction in input from small-diameter afferents leads to a change in pacing during a time trial [80]. Greater muscle activity is produced initially with a consequence of more peripheral fatigue.

In addition to their fatigue sensitivity, small-diameter muscle afferents can also be activated experimentally through injection of hypertonic saline into the muscles. This produces muscle pain. Examination of MEPs and CMEPs in biceps and triceps brachii, with the muscles at rest or during submaximal voluntary contraction, suggests that motoneurones are facilitated while motor cortical excitability is decreased during experimental muscle pain [81]. Maximal voluntary force is reduced and the pattern of motor unit firing is altered [82, 83]. These effects are not wholly consistent with the changes with muscle ischemia after fatigue but small-diameter muscle afferents are not homogeneous and different distributions (and temporal activation) of afferents will occur in the two procedures. Furthermore, the afferents may have different effects on neurones that have not been repetitively active in fatiguing exercise and those that have. Thus, it is not easy to predict the net effect of group III and IV afferents during exercise. However, it seems likely that they act supraspinally to reduce voluntary activation and have more diverse effects at a segmental level.

Conclusion

During exercise of a single limb, the factors that come into play in the development of fatigue are primarily repetitive activation and altered input to muscle fibres and neurones in the motor pathway. At the spinal level, motoneurones fire too slowly to generate maximal possible muscle force. They become more difficult to drive and it is likely that one underlying mechanism is a change in the intrinsic properties of the motoneurones as a result of repetitive activation. For some muscles, inhibition from fatigue-sensitive small-diameter muscle afferents may also contribute, but for other muscles it does not. As well as becoming more difficult to drive, motoneurones may lose excitatory input from muscle spindles in the periphery and/or from descending drive. This is termed disfacilitation. Cortical stimulation can evoke extra motoneuronal output and extra muscle force in the midst of a fatiguing MVC, which indicates that the motoneurones are not completely insensitive to input and could respond to extra excitatory drive. In addition, it indicates that some motor cortical output remains untapped. Thus, output from the motor cortex is suboptimal. However, it is not clear what prevents extra voluntary output from the motor cortex, as the excitability of the motor cortex to stimulation is increased and intracortical inhibition may be decreased. Small-diameter muscle afferents seem to have a role in central fatigue at a cortical level as their activation prevents recovery of supraspinal fatigue and nociceptive afferents decrease excitability of the motor cortex at rest and during submaximal contractions. It is likely that input to the motor cortex from other cortical and subcortical areas is altered but as yet there is no evidence for this.

During whole-body exercise, many other factors will add to the influences of repetitive activation and altered muscle afferent input. These additional factors will impinge on the performance of the motor pathway both through the activation of afferents and through changes in the milieu of the muscle and neurones.

References

[1] Bigland-Ritchie B, Woods JJ. Changes in muscle contractile properties and neural control during human muscular fatigue. *Muscle Nerve*, 1984, 7, 691-9.

[2] Gandevia SC. Spinal and supraspinal factors in human muscle fatigue. *Physiol Rev*, 2001, 81, 1725-89.

[3] Burke RE, Levine DN, Tsairis P, Zajac FE. Physiological types and histochemical profiles in motor units of the cat gastrocnemius. *J Physiol*, 1973, 234, 723-48.

[4] Kernell D, Monster AW. Time course and properties of late adaptation in spinal motoneurones of the cat. *Exp Brain Res*, 1982, 46, 191-6.

[5] Allen DG, Lamb GD, Westerblad H. Skeletal muscle fatigue: Cellular mechanisms. *Physiol Rev*, 2008, 88, 287-332.

[6] Belanger AY, McComas AJ. Extent of motor unit activation during effort. *J Appl Physiol*, 1981, 51, 1131-5.

[7] Merton PA. Voluntary strength and fatigue. *J Physiol*, 1954, 123, 553-64.

[8] Allen GM, Gandevia SC, McKenzie DK. Reliability of measurements of muscle strength and voluntary activation using twitch interpolation. *Muscle Nerve*, 1995, 18, 593-600.

[9] Bigland-Ritchie B, Furbush F, Woods JJ. Fatigue of intermittent submaximal voluntary contractions: Central and peripheral factors. *J Appl Physiol*, 1986, 61, 421-9.

[10] Shield A, Zhou S. Assessing voluntary muscle activation with the twitch interpolation technique. *Sports Med*, 2004, 34, 253-67.

[11] Vagg R, Mogyoros I, Kiernan MC, Burke D. Activity-dependent hyperpolarization of human motor axons produced by natural activity. *J Physiol*, 1998, 507, 919-25.

[12] Jones DA. High- and low-frequency fatigue revisited. *Acta Physiol Scand*, 1996, 156, 265-70.

[13] Martin V, Millet GY, Martin A, Deley G, Lattier G. Assessment of low-frequency fatigue with two methods of electrical stimulation. *J Appl Physiol*, 2004, 97, 1923-9.

[14] Gandevia SC, Allen GM, Butler JE, Taylor JL. Supraspinal factors in human muscle fatigue: Evidence for suboptimal output from the motor cortex. *J Physiol*, 1996, 490, 529-36.

[15] Lee M, Gandevia SC, Carroll TJ. Cortical voluntary activation can be reliably measured in human wrist extensors using transcranial magnetic stimulation. *Clin Neurophysiol*, 2008, 119, 1130-8.

[16] Sidhu SK, Bentley DJ, Carroll TJ. Cortical voluntary activation of the human knee extensors can be reliably estimated using transcranial magnetic stimulation. *Muscle Nerve*, 2009, 39, 186-96.

[17] Todd G, Taylor JL, Gandevia SC. Measurement of voluntary activation of fresh and fatigued human muscles using transcranial magnetic stimulation. *J Physiol*, 2003, 551, 661-71.

[18] Todd G, Taylor JL, Gandevia SC. Reproducible measurement of voluntary activation of human elbow flexors with motor cortical stimulation. *J Appl Physiol*, 2004, 97, 236-42.

[19] Herbert RD, Gandevia SC. Muscle activation in unilateral and bilateral efforts assessed by motor nerve and cortical stimulation. *J Appl Physiol*, 1996, 80, 1351-6.

[20] Thomas CK, Zaidner EY, Calancie B, Broton JG, Bigland-Ritchie BR. Muscle weakness, paralysis, and atrophy after human cervical spinal cord injury. *Exp Neurol*, 1997, 148, 414-23.

[21] Kent-Braun JA. Central and peripheral contributions to muscle fatigue in humans during sustained maximal effort. *Eur J Appl Physiol Occup Physiol*, 1999, 80, 57-63.

[22] Rattey J, Martin PG, Kay D, Cannon J, Marino FE. Contralateral muscle fatigue in human quadriceps muscle: Evidence for a centrally mediated fatigue response and cross-over effect. *Pflugers Arch*, 2005, 452, 1-9.

[23] Schillings ML, Hoefsloot W, Stegeman DF, Zwarts MJ. Relative contributions of central and peripheral factors to fatigue during a maximal sustained effort. *Eur J Appl Physiol*, 2003, 90, 562-8.

[24] Thomas CK, Woods JJ, Bigland-Ritchie B. Impulse propagation and muscle activation in long maximal voluntary contractions. *J Appl Physiol*, 1989, 67, 1835-42.

[25] Sidhu SK, Bentley DJ, Carroll TJ. Locomotor exercise induces long-lasting impairments in the capacity of the human motor cortex to voluntarily activate knee extensor muscles. *J Appl Physiol*, 2009, 106, 556-65.

[26] Todd G, Butler JE, Taylor JL, Gandevia SC. Hyperthermia: A failure of the motor cortex and the muscle. *J Physiol*, 2005, 563, 621-31.

[27] Taylor JL, Todd G, Gandevia SC. Evidence for a supraspinal contribution to human muscle fatigue. *Clin Exp Pharmacol Physiol*, 2006, 33, 400-5.

[28] Nordlund MM, Thorstensson A, Cresswell AG. Central and peripheral contributions to fatigue in relation to level of activation during repeated maximal voluntary isometric plantar flexions. *J Appl Physiol*, 2004, 96, 218-25.

[29] Taylor JL, Allen GM, Butler JE, Gandevia SC. Supraspinal fatigue during intermittent maximal voluntary contractions of the human elbow flexors. *J Appl Physiol*, 2000, 89, 305-13.

[30] McKenzie DK, Bigland-Ritchie B, Gorman RB, Gandevia SC. Central and peripheral fatigue of human diaphragm and limb muscles assessed by twitch interpolation. *J Physiol*, 1992, 454, 643-56.

[31] Kawakami Y, Amemiya K, Kanehisa H, Ikegawa S, Fukunaga T. Fatigue responses of human triceps surae muscles during repetitive maximal isometric contractions. *J Appl Physiol*, 2000, 88, 1969-75.

[32] Löscher WN, Nordlund MM. Central fatigue and motor cortical excitability during repeated shortening and lengthening actions. *Muscle Nerve*, 2002, 25, 864-72.

[33] Adam A, De Luca CJ. Firing rates of motor units in human vastus lateralis muscle during fatiguing isometric contractions. *J Appl Physiol*, 2005, 99, 268-80.

[34] Bigland-Ritchie B, Cafarelli E, Vollestad NK. Fatigue of submaximal static contractions. *Acta Physiol Scand Suppl*, 1986, 556, 137-48.

[35] Smith JL, Martin PG, Gandevia SC, Taylor JL. Sustained contraction at very low forces produces prominent supraspinal fatigue in human elbow flexor muscles. *J Appl Physiol*, 2007, 103, 560-8.

[36] Søgaard K, Gandevia SC, Todd G, Petersen NT, Taylor JL. The effect of sustained low-intensity contractions on supraspinal fatigue in human elbow flexor muscles. *J Physiol*, 2006, 573, 511-23.

[37] Zijdewind I, Zwarts MJ, Kernell D. Influence of a voluntary fatigue test on the contralateral homologous muscle in humans? *Neurosci Lett*, 1998, 253, 41-4.

[38] Taylor JL, Gandevia SC. A comparison of central aspects of fatigue in submaximal and maximal voluntary contractions. *J Appl Physiol*, 2008, 104, 542-50.

[39] Millet GY, Lepers R. Alterations of neuromuscular function after prolonged running, cycling and skiing exercises. *Sports Med*, 2004, 34, 105-16.

[40] Lepers R, Maffiuletti NA, Rochette L, Brugniaux J, Millet GY. Neuromuscular fatigue during a long-duration cycling exercise. *J Appl Physiol*, 2002, 92, 1487-93.

[41] Millet GY, Martin V, Lattier G, Ballay Y. Mechanisms contributing to knee extensor strength loss after prolonged running exercise. *J Appl Physiol*, 2003, 94, 193-8.

[42] Bigland-Ritchie B, Johansson R, Lippold OC, Smith S, Woods JJ. Changes in motoneurone firing rates during sustained maximal voluntary contractions. *J Physiol*, 1983, 340, 335-46.

[43] Gollnick PD, Korge P, Karpakka J, Saltin B. Elongation of skeletal muscle relaxation during exercise is linked to reduced calcium uptake by the sarcoplasmic reticulum in man. *Acta Physiol Scand*, 1991, 142, 135-6.

[44] Todd G, Taylor JL, Butler JE, Martin PG, Gorman RB, Gandevia SC. Use of motor cortex stimulation to measure simultaneously the changes in dynamic muscle

properties and voluntary activation in human muscles. *J Appl Physiol*, 2007, 102, 1756-66.

[45] Kostyukov AI, Bugaychenko LA, Kalezic I, Pilyavskii AI, Windhorst U, Djupsjöbacka M. Effects in feline gastrocnemius-soleus motoneurones induced by muscle fatigue. *Exp Brain Res*, 2005, 163, 284-94.

[46] Macefield G, Hagbarth KE, Gorman R, Gandevia SC, Burke D. Decline in spindle support to alpha-motoneurones during sustained voluntary contractions. *J Physiol*, 440, 497-512.

[47] Pettorossi VE, Torre GD, Bortolami R, Brunetti O. The role of capsaicin-sensitive muscle afferents in fatigue-induced modulation of the monosynaptic reflex in the rat. *J Physiol*, 1999, 515, 599-607.

[48] Jankowska E. Interneuronal relay in spinal pathways from proprioceptors. *Prog Neurobiol*, 1992, 38, 335-78.

[49] Lafleur J, Zytnicki D, Horcholle-Bossavit G, Jami L. Depolarization of Ib afferent axons in the cat spinal cord during homonymous muscle contraction. *J Physiol*, 1992, 445, 345-54.

[50] Zytnicki D, Lafleur J, Horcholle-Bossavit G, Lamy F, Jami L. Reduction of Ib autogenetic inhibition in motoneurons during contractions of an ankle extensor muscle in the cat. *J Neurophysiol*, 1990, 64, 1380-9.

[51] Taylor JL, Gandevia SC. Noninvasive stimulation of the human corticospinal tract. *J Appl Physiol*, 2004, 96, 1496-503.

[52] Ugawa Y, Rothwell JC, Day BL, Thompson PD, Marsden CD. Percutaneous electrical stimulation of corticospinal pathways at the level of the pyramidal decussation in humans. *Ann Neurol*, 1991, 29, 418-27.

[53] Butler JE, Taylor JL, Gandevia SC. Responses of human motoneurons to corticospinal stimulation during maximal voluntary contractions and ischemia. *J Neurosci*, 2003, 23, 10224-30.

[54] Martin PG, Smith JL, Butler JE, Gandevia SC, Taylor JL. Fatigue-sensitive afferents inhibit extensor but not flexor motoneurons in humans. *J Neurosci*, 2006, 26, 4796-802.

[55] Martin PG, Gandevia SC, Taylor JL. Output of human motoneuron pools to corticospinal inputs during voluntary contractions. *J Neurophysiol*, 2006, 95, 3512-8.

[56] Bawa P, Murnaghan C. Motor unit rotation in a variety of human muscles. *J Neurophysiol*, 2009, 102, 2265-72.

[57] Johnson KVB, Edwards SC, Tongeren C, Bawa P. Properties of human motor units after prolonged activity at a constant firing rate. *Exp Brain Res*, 2004, 154, 479-87.

[58] Peters EJD, Fuglevand AJ. Cessation of human motor unit discharge during sustained maximal voluntary contraction. *Neurosci Lett*, 1999, 274, 66-70.

[59] Di Lazzaro V, Oliviero A, Pilato F, Saturno E, Dileone M, Mazzone P, et al. The physiological basis of transcranial motor cortex stimulation in conscious humans. *Clin Neurophysiol*, 2004, 115, 255-66.

[60] Rothwell J, Thompson P, Day B, Boyd S, Marsden C. Stimulation of the human motor cortex through the scalp. *Exp Physiol*, 1991, 76, 159-200.

[61] Siebner HR, Dressnandt J, Auer C, Conrad B. Continuous intrathecal baclofen infusions induced a marked increase of the transcranially evoked silent period in a patient with generalized dystonia. *Muscle Nerve*, 1998, 21, 1209-12.

[62] Werhahn KJ, Kunesch E, Noachtar S, Benecke R, Classen J. Differential effects on motorcortical inhibition induced by blockade of GABA uptake in humans. *J Physiol*, 1999, 517, 591-7.

[63] Taylor JL, Gandevia SC. Transcranial magnetic stimulation and human muscle fatigue. *Muscle Nerve*, 2001, 24, 18-29.

[64] Taylor JL, Butler JE, Allen GM, Gandevia SC. Changes in motor cortical excitability during human muscle fatigue. *J Physiol*, 1996, 490, 519-28.

[65] Liu JZ, Dai TH, Sahgal V, Brown RW, Yue GH. Nonlinear cortical modulation of muscle fatigue: A functional MRI study. *Brain Res*, 2002, 957, 320-9.

[66] Benwell N, Mastaglia F, Thickbroom G. Differential changes in long-interval intracortical inhibition and silent period duration during fatiguing hand exercise. *Exp Brain Res*, 2007, 179, 255-62.

[67] Benwell N, Sacco P, Hammond G, Byrnes M, Mastaglia F, Thickbroom G. Short-interval cortical inhibition and corticomotor excitability with fatiguing hand exercise: A central adaptation to fatigue? *Exp Brain Res*, 2006, 170, 191-8.

[68] Maruyama A, Matsunaga K, Tanaka N, Rothwell JC. Muscle fatigue decreases short-interval intracortical inhibition after exhaustive intermittent tasks. *Clin Neurophysiol*, 2006, 117, 864-70.

[69] McNeil CJ, Martin PG, Gandevia SC, Taylor JL. The response to paired motor cortical stimuli is abolished at a spinal level during human muscle fatigue. *J Physiol*, 2009, 587, 5601-12.

[70] Kniffki KD, Schomburg ED, Steffens H. Synaptic responses of lumbar alpha-motoneurones to chemical algesic stimulation of skeletal muscle in spinal cats. *Brain Res*, 1979, 160, 549-52.

[71] Li J, Sinoway LI. ATP stimulates chemically sensitive and sensitizes mechanically sensitive afferents. *Am J Physiol Heart Circ Physiol*, 2002, 283, H2636-43.

[72] Mense S. Nervous outflow from skeletal muscle following chemical noxious stimulation. *J Physiol*, 1977, 267, 75-88.

[73] Rotto DM, Kaufman MP. Effect of metabolic products of muscular contraction on discharge of group III and IV afferents. *J Appl Physiol*, 1988, 64, 2306-13.

[74] Sinoway LI, Hill JM, Pickar JG, Kaufman MP. Effects of contraction and lactic acid on the discharge of group III muscle afferents in cats. *J Neurophysiol*, 1993, 69, 1053-9.

[75] Garland SJ. Role of small diameter afferents in reflex inhibition during human muscle fatigue. *J Physiol*, 1991, 435, 547-58.

[76] Woods JJ, Furbush F, Bigland-Ritchie B. Evidence for a fatigue-induced reflex inhibition of motoneuron firing rates. *J Neurophysiol*, 1987, 58, 125-37.

[77] Garland SJ, McComas AJ. Reflex inhibition of human soleus muscle during fatigue. *J Physiol*, 1990, 429, 17-27.

[78] Rossi A, Decchi B, Ginanneschi F. Presynaptic excitability changes of group Ia fibres to muscle nociceptive stimulation in humans. *Brain Res*, 1999, 818, 12-22.

[79] Taylor JL, Petersen N, Butler JE, Gandevia SC. Ischaemia after exercise does not reduce responses of human motoneurones to cortical or corticospinal tract stimulation. *J Physiol*, 2000, 525, 793-801.

[80] Amann M, Proctor LT, Sebranek JJ, Pegelow DF, Dempsey JA. Opioid-mediated muscle afferents inhibit central motor drive and limit peripheral muscle fatigue development in humans. *J Physiol*, 2009, 587, 271-83.

[81] Martin PG, Weerakkody N, Gandevia SC, Taylor JL. Group III and IV muscle afferents differentially affect the motor cortex and motoneurones in humans. *J Physiol*, 2008, 586, 1277-89.

[82] Graven-Nielsen T, Svensson P, Arendt-Nielsen L. Effects of experimental muscle pain on muscle activity and co-ordination during static and dynamic motor function. *Electroencephalogr Clin Neurophysiol*, 1997, 105, 156-64.

[83] Tucker K, Butler J, Graven-Nielsen T, Riek S, Hodges P. Motor unit recruitment strategies are altered during deep-tissue pain. *J Neurosci*, 2009, 29, 10820-6.

In: Regulation of Fatigue in Exercise
Editor: Frank E. Marino

ISBN 978-1-61209-334-5

Chapter 5

THE VO_{2MAX} AND THE CENTRAL GOVERNOR: A DIFFERENT UNDERSTANDING

Timothy David Noakes
UCT/MRC Research Unit for Exercise Science and Sports Medicine, Department of Human Biology, University of Cape Town and Sports Science Institute of South Africa, Boundary Road, Newlands, 7700, South Africa

ABSTRACT

In 1923, Nobel Laureate A.V. Hill introduced his cardiovascular/ anaerobic/ catastrophic model of human exercise performance. According to this model, maximal exercise testing for the measurement of the maximum oxygen consumption (VO_2max) terminates when the maximum rate of oxygen delivery to the exercising muscles is less than their peak rate of oxygen demand. As a result skeletal muscle anaerobiosis develops, causing fatigue and the termination of exercise. The weakness of this interpretation is that it is "brainless" since it excludes any role for the brain in determining maximal exercise performance. Yet without the brain, there can be no skeletal muscle recruitment, without which exercise cannot occur. The analogy is a racing car: A racing car filled with petrol will not move off the starting grid until the brain of the racing driver starts the car's engine, engages first gear and applies pressure to the car's accelerator. The role of the brain in exercise performance is identical; until the muscles are recruited by the motor cortex, they will not function; without increasing skeletal muscle recruitment, the oxygen consumption and cardiac output cannot rise. Thus it is the level of skeletal muscle recruitment that must determine the athlete's maximal work rate as well as the extent to which the cardiac output and oxygen consumption rise during the VO_2max test. Remarkably the Hill model has instilled the reverse doctrine specifically that the cardiac output, not the level of skeletal muscle recruitment, determines the work output of the muscles. In this chapter I present 6 biological predictions of the Hill model of maximal exercise performance that have been disproven specifically that (i) the "plateau phenomenon" does not occur in 100% of subjects during VO_2max testing; (ii) skeletal muscle anaerobiosis does not occur during maximal exercise; (iii) the cardiac output does not show a "plateau phenomenon" nor (iv) are all available motor units activated in the exercising limbs of all subjects during VO_2max testing; (v) fatigue does not always develop at the same level of "fatiguing" metabolites; and (vi) fatigue is never absolute. Instead the evidence is that the VO_2max test is a submaximal test that is terminated by the brain when less than 100% of the motor units in the exercising limbs have been recruited. The protected variable that triggers this anticipatory termination of the VO_2 max test is currently unknown but may well relate to changes in cerebral oxygenation.

INTRODUCTION

On the basis of his interpretation that fatigue is caused by anaerobiosis in the exercising muscles as a result of the development of myocardial ischaemia, in 1923 Professor Archibald Vivian Hill introduced the concept of the maximum oxygen consumption (VO_2max) into the exercise sciences (Chapter 1). In 1955 H.L. Taylor and colleagues[1] established this concept by stating that: "The classic work of Hill has demonstrated that there is an upper limit to the capacity of the combined respiratory and cardiovascular systems to transport oxygen to the muscles. There is a linear relationship between oxygen intake and work rate until the maximum oxygen intake is reached. Further increases in workload beyond this point merely result in an increase in oxygen debt and a shortening of the time in which the work can be performed".

These scientists were also the first to describe the concept that would become known as the "plateau phenomenon": "Each day the (running) speed was increased until the oxygen uptake during the standard collection time reached a plateau". In the past 50 years few have felt it necessary to question the veracity of these concepts. Those who have dared[2-5], have usually attracted a dismissive response[5-15] suggesting that new ideas are not always welcome in the exercise sciences.

In a recent publication Mitchell and Saltin[16] provided their most current interpretation of Hill's contribution to our understanding of the physiological basis for the VO_2max: "It is noteworthy that although well-designed treadmills were available, Hill preferred walking and running in the field or on the track for his experiments. To determine the velocity of the runner, he developed a sophisticated electromagnetic system that provided split times for every 25 yards. In the experiments on Hill himself, a levelling off in VO_2 was observed, not as a function of increasing speed of running, but with the time at the highest velocity, which was 260 meters.min^{-1}[17]. Noakes has challenged whether Hill actually demonstrated a plateau in VO_2 and thus had measured a true VO_2max[3]. Hill appears to have accomplished this in the experiments conducted on himself; but more importantly, he was the one who conceived the physiological meaning of maximal VO_2."

Elsewhere [18, 19] I have provided the contradictory evidence which shows that Hill was absolutely convinced that his model of the physiological factors limiting the VO_2max was beyond doubt. So why would he have considered it necessary to "prove" this theory by showing the presence of the "plateau phenomenon"? In his mind he had already done that. Only later, when his theory began to be questioned for the first time, did a modern generation of scientists feel the urgent need to "prove" that Hill's ideas were correct by attempting to show that the "plateau phenomenon" or some equivalent [10, 11, 15, 20, 21] always causes the termination of exercise in all VO_2max tests (as is required by the Hill model).

In fact, as argued in Chapter 1, the real test of a maximal effort according to the Hill model must be the development of myocardial ischaemia and cardiac failure, according to Hill's idea that: "When the oxygen supply becomes inadequate, it is probable that the heart rapidly begins to diminish its output, so avoiding exhaustion"[22].

However the well-established finding that myocardial ischaemia does not occur during maximal exercise in healthy subjects [23] disproves this component of Hill's model. Not surprisingly protagonists of this model chose to ignore this inconvenient finding, continuing rather to argue that it is the presence of a "plateau phenomenon", defined in at least 10 different ways [24] that proves the model. Whereas I argue that according to the Hill model the sole proof that a VO_2max test is "truly maximal" is the development of myocardial ischaemia. Or alternatively that exercise terminates only after all the available motor units in the active limbs have been recruited (Chapter 1).

Mitchell and Saltin[16] included a diagram, redrawn here as Figure 1, which explained why they believe the VO_2max is limited by the maximum cardiac output and the maximum systemic arterio-venous oxygen difference. According to this (Hill) model, three factors, namely cardiovascular function (specifically the maximum cardiac output), the blood haemoglobin concentration, and the extent to which oxygen is extracted from the arterial blood by the active muscles determine the magnitude of the VO_2max. The focus of this chapter is to argue that the model depicted in Figure 1 is only valid if exercise is indeed limited by a failure of oxygen delivery to the exercising muscles as Hill had presumed in 1923 but which, I argue, his data did not ever prove [4, 18, 24, 25].

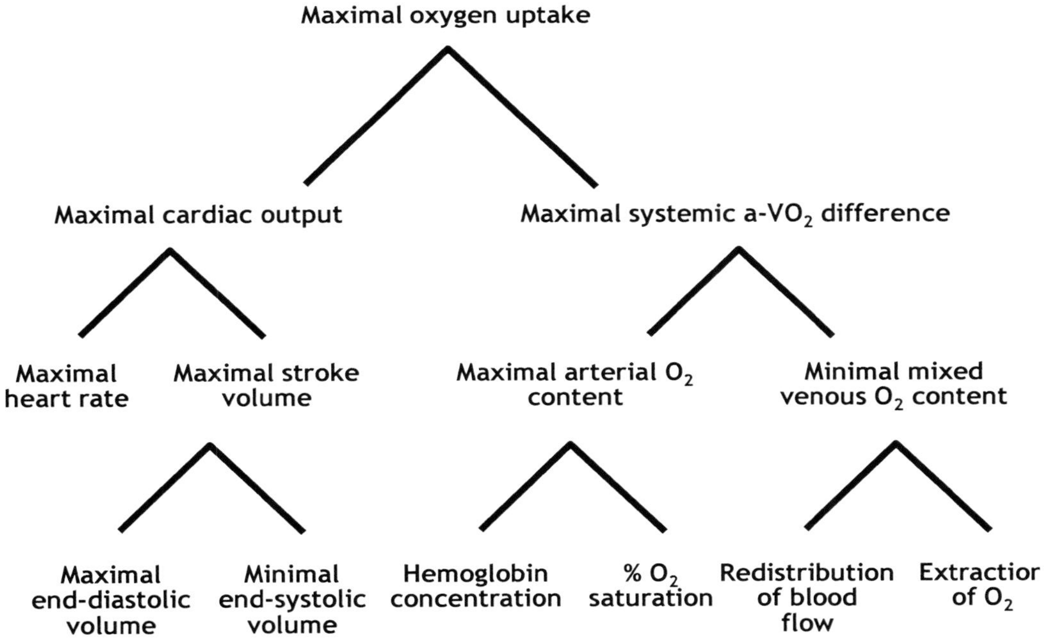

Figure 1. The physiological factors that determine or "limit" the maximum oxygen consumption (VO_2max) according to the traditional A.V. Hill model. After Mitchell and Saltin [16].

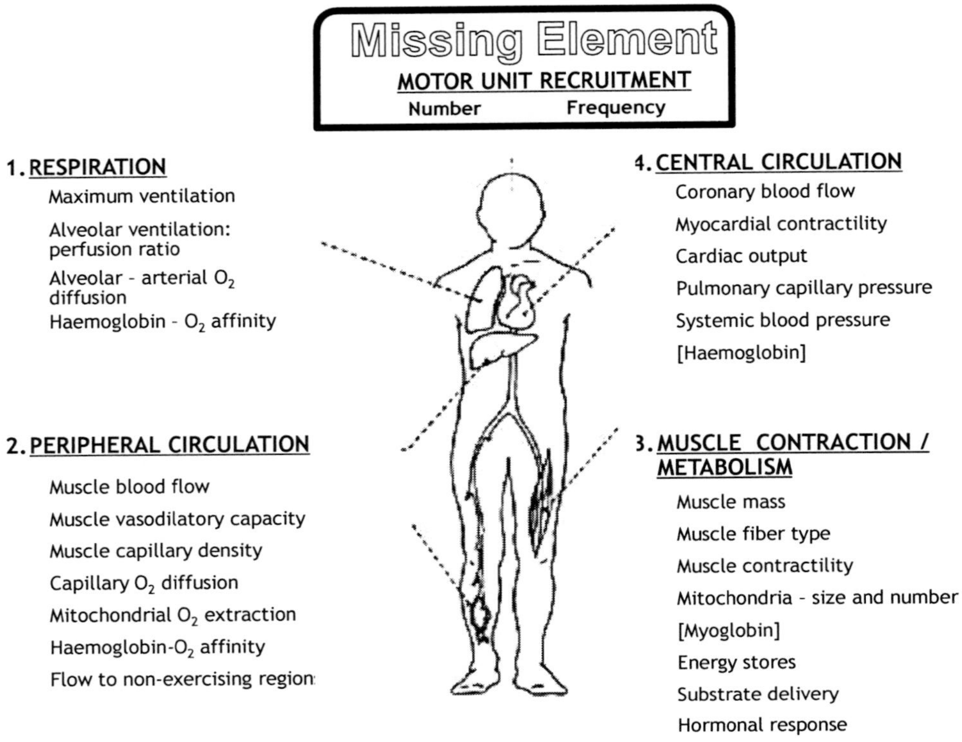

Figure 2. The popular diagram showing the four physiological systems (respiration, peripheral circulation, central circulation and muscle contraction/metabolism) that are believed to "limit" the VO_2max according to the traditional A.V. Hill model. The missing element in this diagram is the central nervous system. Without the recruitment of sufficient motor units in the limbs, movement and hence exercise is not possible. Without an increased skeletal muscle recruitment, there can be no increase in VO_2. In which case the "VO_2max" is limited by the absence of the brain.

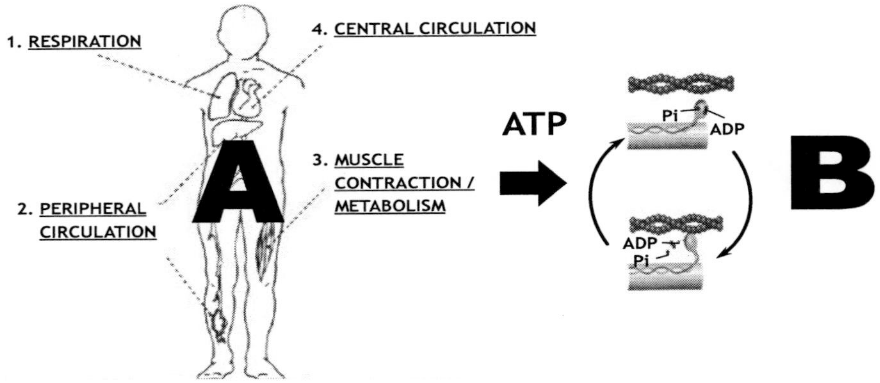

Figure 3. According to the Hill model the function of the cardiorespiratory system and skeletal muscle metabolism (A) is to maximize the rate of ATP production (B) so that the rate of force production by the muscle is also maximal.

The core belief of the Hill model is that the capacity of the heart and cardiovascular system to provide oxygen to the exercising muscles determines the exercise performance. As P.O. Astrand wrote in his PhD thesis in 1952: "The working capacity of the heart may determine that of the muscles" [26]. Or as Levine has written more recently: "the primary distinguishing characteristic of elite endurance athletes that allows them to run fast over prolonged periods of time is a large, compliant heart with a compliant pericardium that can accommodate a lot of blood, very fast, to take advantage of the Starling mechanism to generate a large stroke volume"[6] (p. 31).

This theory has been expanded somewhat into a popular diagram (Figure 2) which proposes that factors relating to respiration, peripheral circulation, central circulation and muscle metabolism ultimately determine human exercise capacity. According to this theory, the key function of these systems is to ensure that there is a maximal rate of ATP generation in the muscles.

As a consequence it is believed that the critical determinant of the amount of work that the muscles can perform is the rate at which the cardio-respiratory and metabolic systems (A) can supply ATP (B) to fuel the actin and myosin cross-bridge cycles in the exercising muscles (Figure 3). But the ignored elephant in this particular sitting room is the absence of the brain. For without the brain, the depicted human would be unable to stand, let alone exercise vigorously. An intriguing question is: Why has it taken so long for anyone to detect the obvious omission from this diagram?

Figure 4 explains why this model cannot be the truth. For the simple reason that the provision of ATP does not activate the cross-bridge cycle; rather something more than just ATP is required to induce a muscle contraction (which can then utilize the ATP so generously provided by these other systems). The analogy might be to a racing car that has a full tank of petrol. Even with a full tank a racing car cannot begin the race unless a driver starts the engine, engages first gear and applies his foot forcibly to the accelerator.

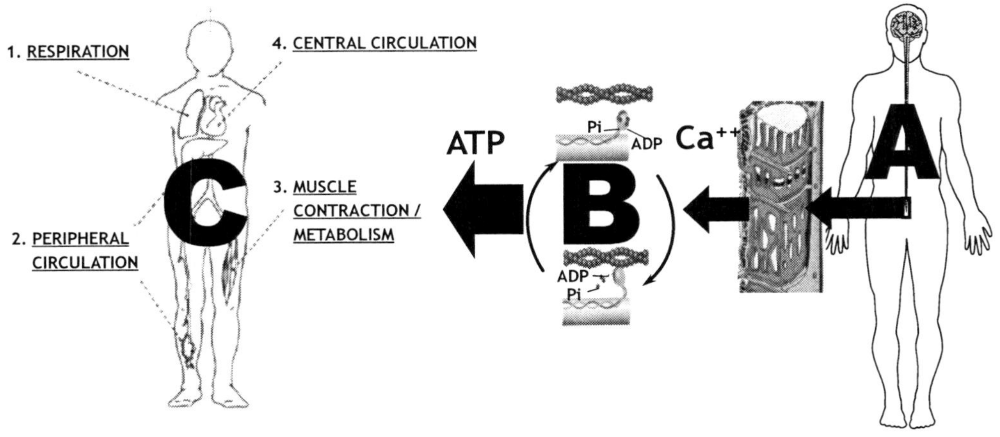

Figure 4. Skeletal muscle contraction (B) is initiated by calcium release from the sarcoplasmic reticulum which is dependent on the functioning of intact central and peripheral nervous systems (A). The cardiorespiratory and skeletal muscle metabolic systems (C) function to generate ATP at rates sufficient to cover the demands generated by skeletal muscle recruitment directed by the central nervous system.

In the analogy to skeletal muscle contraction, the driver is the central nervous system (Figure 4). His action in pressing the accelerator is equivalent to the neurally-regulated release of calcium from the sarcoplasmic reticulum within the muscle fibers. The arrival of calcium at the myofilaments allows the cross-bridge cycle to occur; only then is ATP required (in proportion to the number of cross-bridges that are formed) to allow each cross-bridge to relax before another cross-bridge can be formed. Thus the amount of ATP required to sustain this activity is a function of the exercising workload. But it is **not** the ATP that drives muscle contraction.

The analogy is complete when it is realized that the function of the driver's brain is to ensure that the racing car completes the race safely without driving so fast that it leaves the race track destroying the car and potentially also the driver. The brain does this by always insuring that it recruits just sufficient motor units (and hence muscle fibers) in the driver's right calf muscles so that the pressure on the accelerator always produces the correct car speed, appropriate for each segment of the race track and for each moment of the race.

The Central Governor Model (CGM) predicts that during exercise the brain acts identically, insuring that just sufficient motor units are always activated in the exercising limbs to ensure that the exercise can be completed safely. The brain achieves this by modifying behavior in anticipation to ensure that the brain, the body and ultimately the human species survive. The brain of the athlete, like that of the racing car driver, is interested ultimately in survival. As a result all athletic performances are submaximal since the only truly maximal athletic performance would be the one that causes the athlete's death.

As a result, the missing factor in the traditional diagram of the factors limiting exercise performance is the role of the brain in directing the extent of skeletal muscle recruitment on a moment-to-moment basis during exercise. I argue that the goal of this control must be to insure the protection of whole body homeostasis.

The Six Physiological Predictions of the A.V. Hill Model

Two key concepts in science are that (i) we can interpret scientific information, including new data, only according to a conceptual model of how we think a particular system works. The value of these models is that they make predictions which can then be tested in appropriate experiments. But (ii) a conceptual model must be changed as soon as evidence that it does not predict becomes available. Once there is even a single finding that is not predicted by a particular model, that model must be either modified or discarded, or else it becomes a "creaking and ugly edifice" [3]. It is my contention that the A.V. Hill model makes at least 6 predictions, all of which have been disproven. As a result, I continue to argue that the A.V. Hill model needs to be retired and replaced by a model that better explains all (not just some) of the relevant findings in the exercise sciences. The six predictions of the A.V. Hill cardiovascular/anaerobic/catastrophic (CAC) model (Chapter 1) that in our view [24] have been disproven are the following:

First Disproven Prediction of A.V. Hill's CAC Model

A stable, non-rising "plateau phenomenon" does not occur in 100% of subjects causing termination of the VO_2 Max test.

Hill's explanation of the physiological events that cause the termination of maximal exercise was, as described in the companion chapter (Figure 4 in Chapter 1), unambiguous. He believed that the development of myocardial ischemia, limited by a governor that protected the heart by reducing acutely its pumping capacity, led to skeletal muscle anaerobiosis, lactic acidosis and the impairment of skeletal muscle relaxation.

Since this description is so precise, it should be easily detectable by the following sequence of events: (i) The development of acute myocardial ischaemia with the diagnostic symptoms of angina pectoris followed by (ii) an abrupt plateau in cardiac output and in oxygen consumption (VO_2), leading to (iii) a fall in cardiac output and VO_2 as progressive cardiac failure develops consequent to (iv) continuing myocardial ischaemia.

But the reality is that the only "evidence" for this sequence of events is that, in a certain proportion of tested subjects, the VO_2 does not increase linearly up to the point of exercise termination. This classic response was depicted in the highly influential paper by Mitchell and Blomqvist published in the New England Journal of Medicine in 1971 (Figure 5; see also Figure 2 in Chapter 1). These figures suggest that the oxygen consumption exhibits the "plateau phenomenon" for at least 2 workloads before the termination of any bout of progressive maximal exercise.

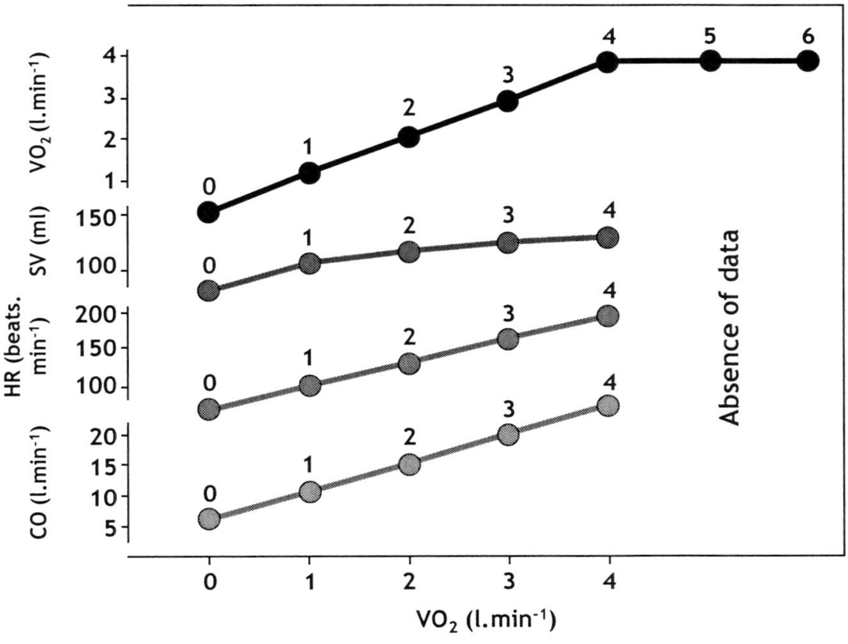

Figure 5. An original diagram [55] of the cardiovascular changes during exercise up to the point at which the VO_2max is achieved failed to indicate the changes in stroke volume, heart rate and cardiac output that, according to the Hill model, must occur subsequent to the achievement of VO_2max.

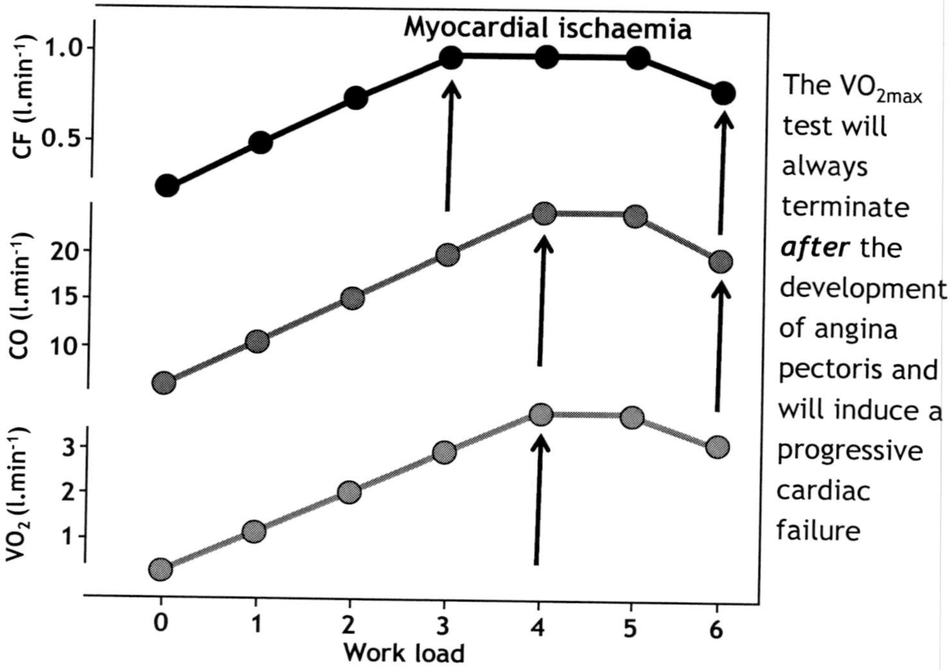

Figure 6. If the cardiac output limits the VO_2max, then this must be because there is first a plateau in coronary blood flow which induces myocardial ischaemia, angina pectoris and a progressive cardiac failure followed by a falling VO_2.

It is interesting that the text accompanying that figure makes no reference to the changes in cardiovascular function that must happen once the "plateau phenomenon" has occurred. In a previous paper[4] I argued that the cause of the plateau in VO_2 must be a plateau in cardiac output caused by a plateau in coronary blood flow leading to myocardial ischaemia and a progressive cardiac failure (Figure 6). According to this interpretation, faithful to Hill's original interpretation, the VO_2max test must always terminate *after* the development of myocardial ischaemia, angina pectoris and a progressive cardiac failure (Chapter 1).

One of the more interesting studies that has relevance to this theory is shown in Figure 7. In that study [20] the change in VO_2 immediately preceding the termination of the test was studied in approximately 70 subjects. In 28% of the tests, the subjects' VO_2 rose exponentially immediately prior to the termination of the test (Figure 7; top panel). In another 55% of tests, the subjects' VO_2 rose linearly up to the point of exhaustion (Figure 7; middle panel). In only 12 subjects, that is in only 17% of the total study population, did the VO_2 appear to reach a "plateau" prior to the termination of exercise (Figure 7; bottom panel). The authors did not report that any test terminated after the development of myocardial ischaemia and angina pectoris.

Thus these data provided by a group with a strong belief that the VO_2max is determined by a failure of oxygen delivery to the muscles [20, 21, 27], found that more than 80% of these maximal exercise tests terminated without any evidence for a "plateau phenomenon", however liberally defined. According to the logic applied by A.V. Hill, this finding must mean that more than 80% of these tests did ***not*** terminate as a result of skeletal muscle anaerobiosis consequent to the development of a maximal cardiac output and myocardial ischaemia. But instead of acknowledging this inconvenient truth, the authors spun the finding as evidence that it is unnecessary to demonstrate the "plateau phenomenon" to prove that a "true" VO_2max had been achieved.

As one of the reviewers of that paper I encouraged the authors to add some discussion of how their data disprove this key prediction of the A.V. Hill model. Not unsurprisingly the authors were allowed to publish their paper in one of the world's leading journals of physiology without any reference to this important conclusion, which must indicate that there is a publication bias favoring those articles that appear to support the predictions of the A.V. Hill model.

In our review [24] of the limitations of the A.V. Hill model, we analyzed 33 studies that have reported the percentage of VO_2max tests that terminated with or without evidence for a "plateau phenomenon". Considering that the physiological events causing the "plateau phenomenon" are supposed to be absolutely specific (Figure 4 in Chapter 1) – the development of a maximum cardiac output leading to an *abrupt* failure of oxygen delivery to the exercising muscles – it is surprising that there are at least 10 different definitions of how these events can be identified. Of a total of 1978 individual VO_2max tests reported in the literature by 2004, 44% showed evidence for some form of "plateau phenomenon" as defined by one or more of these 10 different criteria.

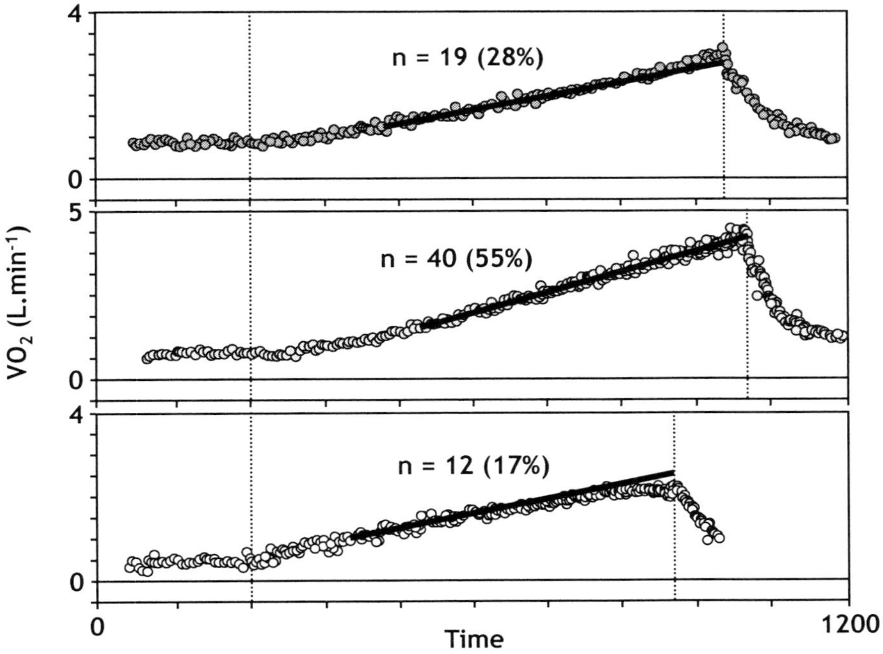

Figure 7. The study of Day et al. [20] found that there were 3 different patterns of change in VO_2 preceding the termination of exercise during testing for the VO_2max. In 28% of subjects (top panel) the VO_2 rose exponentially immediately prior to exercise termination; in 55% the rise was linear (middle panel) and in only 17% was there evidence for a "plateau phenomenon" (bottom panel).

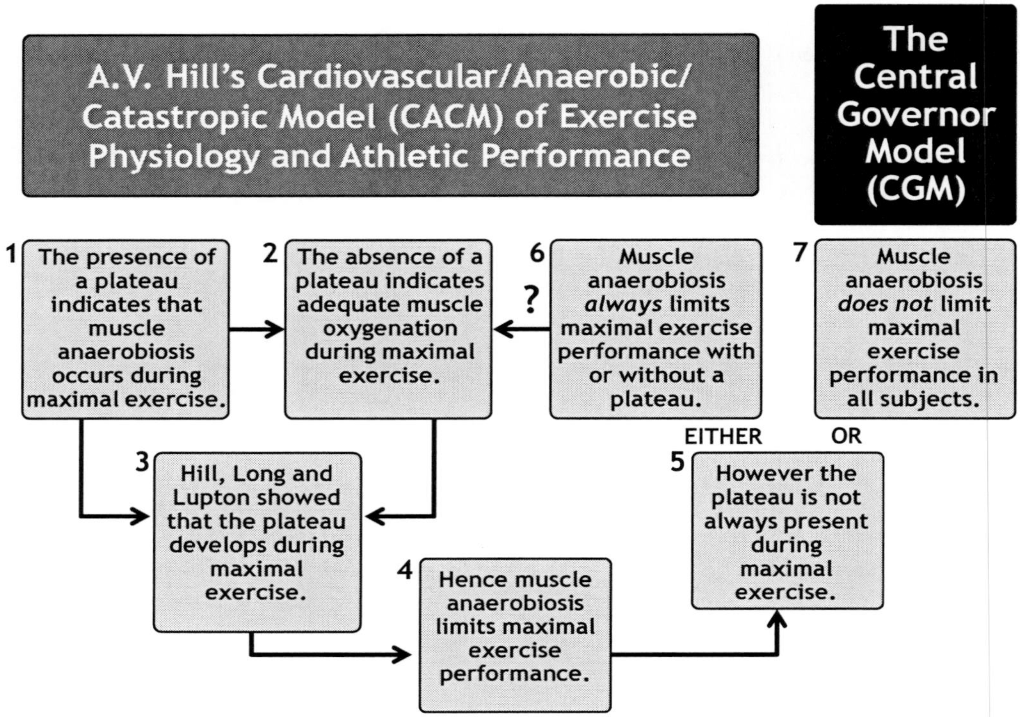

Figure 8. If skeletal muscle anaerobiosis identified by the presence of the "plateau" phenomenon causes the termination of exercise, then the absence of this phenomenon in some must indicate that factors other than skeletal muscle anaerobiosis cause the termination of exercise in those subjects.

Aside from the obvious comment that a physiological event which is supposed to be so specific should produce a characteristic and easily identifiable physiological response, specifically an *abrupt* ceiling in the rate of whole body VO_2 measured by sampling the expired air, this finding raises an even more important question: What causes the termination of exercise in the ~50% of subjects who do not show any evidence for a "plateau phenomenon", however defined, immediately prior to the termination of the VO_2max test? According to the predictions of the A.V. Hill model, this cannot be due to a limiting cardiac output, skeletal muscle anaerobiosis, lactic acidosis and a failure of skeletal muscle relaxation. But if these (patho) physiological changes do not cause the termination of exercise, then the obvious question is: What does?

Figure 8 first published in 1998 and since largely ignored, compares the interpretation of these data according to either the A.V. Hill model or the CGM. The key argument is that the ***absence*** of a "plateau phenomenon" must indicate the ***presence*** of adequate muscle oxygenation during maximal exercise. For if this is not true, then neither is the converse. And if the converse is not true, then the A.V.Hill model is not valid.

Thus if a "plateau" is not present at the termination of a VO_2max test, then the cause of that exercise termination cannot be explained by the A.V. Hill model since that model requires that myocardial failure and skeletal muscle anaerobiosis must always occur before the exercise terminates. In contrast, the CGM explains the absence of the "plateau phenomenon" as evidence that a factor or factors other than skeletal muscle anaerobiosis must cause the termination of maximal exercise in those subjects.

According to the CGM, the presence of the "plateau phenomenon" could be explained by a number of phenomena other than simply the development of skeletal muscle anaerobiosis. For example, it could indicate an increased reliance on oxygen-independent metabolism in anticipation that the exercise is about to terminate (so that there is no need to further increase oxygen utilization). This fits with the idea that the central governor has the capacity to act in an anticipatory manner (Chapter 1).

Second Disproven Prediction

Skeletal muscle anaerobiosis does not occur during maximal exercise in humans.

The second absolute prediction of the A.V. Hill model is that skeletal muscle anaerobiosis must be present at exhaustion in 100% of subjects. Remarkably, two of the leading scientists studying skeletal muscle oxygenation during maximal exercise have both concluded that skeletal muscle anaerobiosis does not occur during maximal exercise even when maximal exercise is performed in hypoxia.

Thus in 1998 Richardson and colleagues [28] concluded that: "...skeletal muscle cells do not become anaerobic ... since intracellular PO_2 is well preserved at a constant level even at maximal exercise" and that "average intracellular PO_2 remains above PO_{2crit} even at maximal exercise in hypoxia". Similarly, Mole et al. [29] concluded that: "...O_2 availability is not limiting VO_2 during exercise". Perhaps not surprisingly these inconvenient conclusions of such leading scientists have been ignored since they disprove the foundation belief on which A.V. Hill built his model.

Instead what seems to be favored is that which Fletcher and Hopkins [30] (Chapter 1) wrote in 1907: "Lactic acid is spontaneously developed under anaerobic conditions...".

Third Disproven Prediction

The cardiac output does not show a "plateau phenomenon" in 100% of subjects at the termination of the VO_2 Max test.

The third absolute requirement of the A.V. Hill model is that the cardiac output must *always* be maximal at fatigue since the heart is merely the slave to the oxygen demands of the exercising muscles. As a consequence the heart must pump to its maximum capacity whenever fatigue occurs in order to maximize oxygen delivery to the oxygen-starved muscles. But a number of studies have established that exercise frequently terminates before the cardiac output or stroke volume reaches a "plateau" or maximum value[31]. The notable exceptions are a series of studies many from the same laboratory, which show a plateau in cardiac output during high-intensity exercise [32]. In contrast scientists from another laboratory who consistently argue that oxygen limits exercise performance [33-35] are unable to find a plateau in cardiac output during maximal exercise [36]. Yet they nevertheless still conclude that "in healthy humans VO_2max is limited by cardiac output and skeletal muscle blood flow".

But if the cardiac output does indeed "plateau" during maximal exercise, then this should cause myocardial ischaemia as it does in persons with coronary artery stenosis [37], for the reasons described in Chapter 1. None of the subjects in the studies apparently showing a "plateau" in cardiac output reported the development of angina pectoris which must occur if cardiac output reaches a true maximum. In one study the central venous pressure reportedly rose [38]. This is surprising since this indicates the onset of cardiac failure. Yet if cardiac failure is indeed the reason why maximal exercise terminates in young, healthy subjects, as predicted by the A.V. Hill model, then surely other researchers would also have reported that finding sometime in the past 80 years?

However the most striking and well documented example of a failure to achieve a maximum cardiac output at exercise termination occurs during maximal exercise in extreme hypoxia. Under those conditions the well-described "lactate paradox" of high altitude (hypoxia) occurs [39]. In this condition, blood lactate concentrations are low at exhaustion. Less well appreciated is the "cardiac output paradox" of high altitude in which both the cardiac output and heart rate are also sub-maximal at exhaustion.

A popular explanation is that the heart becomes progressively more hypoxic at increasing altitude; its function fails [40] and, as a consequence, it is unable to provide enough oxygen to the exercising muscles. But there is clear evidence that the heart is not hypoxic during maximum exercise at altitude [33, 34, 41-43]; thus this explanation whilst convenient, is simply wrong. A more likely explanation [39] is that the extent of skeletal muscle recruitment becomes progressively less at increasing altitude [44] or increasing levels of induced hypoxia[45] so that paradoxically low cardiac outputs and blood lactate concentrations are simply the result of reduced levels of skeletal muscle recruitment allowed by the brain at increasing altitude or greater levels of hypoxia.

The finding that the "maximal" cardiac output in hypoxia is sub-maximal is especially paradoxical according to the A.V. Hill model. This is because the cardiac output should be as high or higher during maximum exercise in hypoxia than in normoxia so that the delivery of blood with a lower oxygen content can be maximized. Rather the more reasonable explanation is that skeletal muscle recruitment is reduced at altitude; this reduces the oxygen demands of the exercising muscles as well as the rates of skeletal muscle lactate production and release.

Figure 9 explains why I think so many find it difficult to understand this paradox. This figure shows the cardiac output/work rate relationship in an experiment reported by Calbet and colleagues [34]. The traditional (Hill) method of interpreting this figure is to assume that the cardiac output drives the work rate; in other words that A, a greater cardiac output, causes B, the higher work rate. But the CGM argues that it is the brain's feed-forward recruitment (C) of the motor units in the exercising limbs that determines the work rate, the oxygen demand of the exercising muscles and hence the cardiac output (A). According to this interpretation, the cardiac output does not determine the work rate. Rather the level to which the cardiac output rises is determined by the passive cardiovascular response to the oxygen demands of the tissues. This demand is in turn determined by the motor cortex as part of a complex feed-forward control mechanism. This is the CGM.

Thus if the cardiac output is low at exhaustion, it is because the level of skeletal muscle recruitment is also low. This is the key interpretation that devotees of the Hill model have great difficulty understanding.

Fourth Disproven Prediction

All available motor units are never activated in the exercising limbs at exhaustion.

The fourth absolute requirement of the A.V. Hill model is that complete recruitment of all available motor units in the active limbs must occur some time prior to the development of exhaustion. For unless there is complete skeletal muscle recruitment at exhaustion during voluntary exercise, the central nervous system must be regulating that performance.

For the clear prediction of the A.V. Hill model must be that as each motor unit becomes fatigued, the brain is forced to recruit additional units to sustain the activity. Ultimately when fatigue develops in the final motor unit recruited, the force output of the active muscles must also fall causing the exercise to terminate.

In contrast, the CGM predicts that motor unit recruitment is regulated and never maximal so that exercise always terminates before there is a maximal skeletal muscle recruitment. Already in 1997 Sloniger and colleagues [46, 47] showed that muscle activation was not maximal in any of the major lower limb muscle groups at exhaustion during maximal horizontal or uphill running. This has since been confirmed in a study [48] which found that in none of the lower limb muscle groups was muscle activation at exhaustion during a VO_2max test more than about 70% of that achieved during a short bout of maximal sprint cycling (Figure 10).

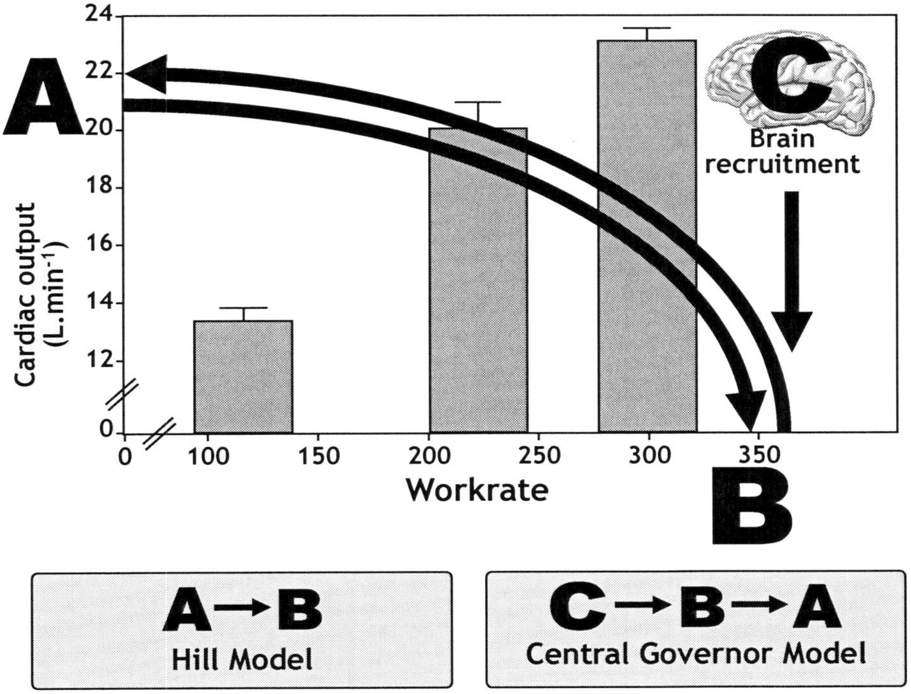

Figure 9. The Hill model predicts that it is the increase in cardiac output (A) that produces the increase in work rate (B) that occurs during progressive exercise to exhaustion. In contrast the Central Governor Model predicts that an increased motor command from the brain determines the increase in work rate that occurs during this form of exercise. The greater power output produced by the increased number of motor units that are activated in the exercising limbs, increases the blood and oxygen demands of the active skeletal muscles. As a consequence the cardiac output rises (C).

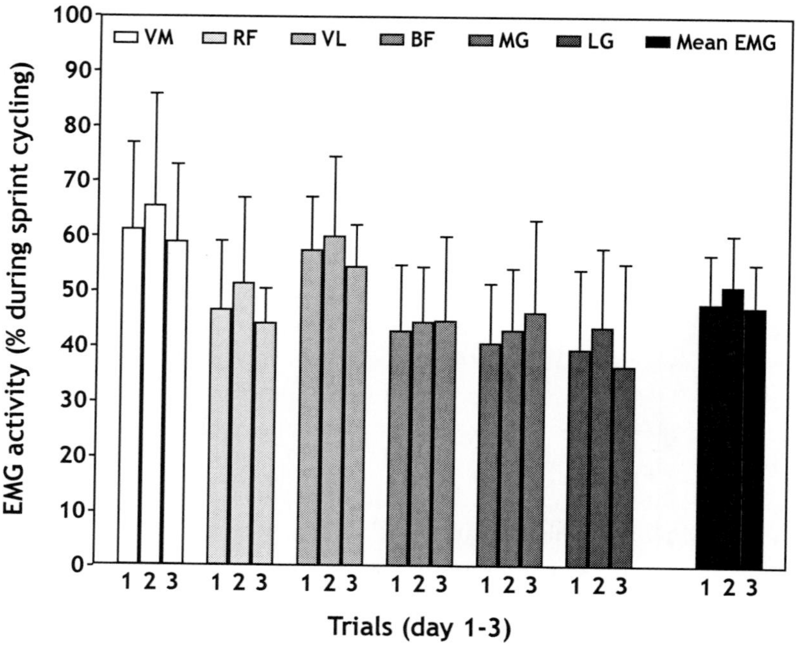

Figure 10. The study of Albertus[48] showed that the level of skeletal muscle recruitment in 6 different muscle groups during VO_2max testing averaged about 50% of that achieved during a short burst of maximal cycling exercise. VM vastus medialis; RF rectus femoris; VL vastus lateralis; BF biceps femoris; MG medial gastrocnemius; LG lateral gastrocnemius; EMG electromyography.

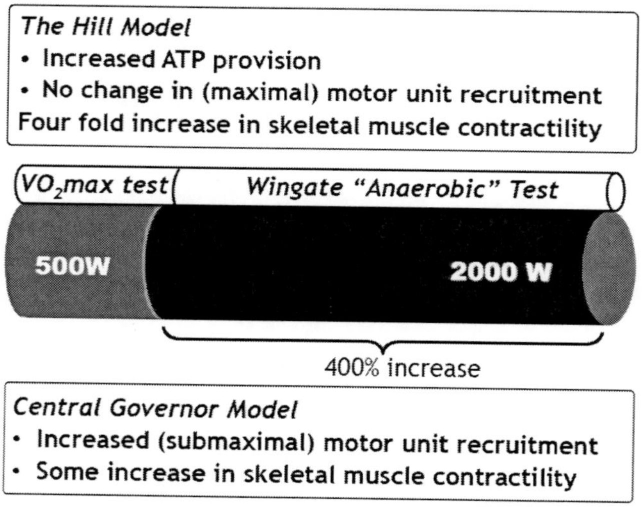

Figure 11. The Hill model requires that the 4-fold higher "maximal" power output during a Wingate "Anaerobic" test (2000W) than during a VO_2max test (400W), must be due to 4-fold increase in muscle contractility without any increase in skeletal muscle recruitment. In contrast the Central Governor Model predicts that this increase in "maximal" power output is more likely explained by a much greater level of skeletal muscle recruitment during the Wingate "Anaerobic" test than during the VO_2max test with perhaps a small change in skeletal muscle contractility.

Figure 11 depicts the explanations provided by either the A.V. Hill model or the CGM of the factors explaining exercise performance during either short duration exercise of very high intensity or during a VO_2max test. The A.V. Hill model predicts that at the point of exhaustion during the VO_2max test all motor units are active since the exercise must terminate only after "peripheral fatigue" has developed in all the available muscle fibers (motor units) in the exercising limbs.

But this explanation seems unlikely since there are no known mechanisms by which skeletal muscle fibers can increase their contractility fourfold. Nor would it seem logical that this contractility "reserve" is activated only during "anaerobic" exercise of very short duration and not during more prolonged maximal "aerobic" exercise. In contrast, the CGM predicts that a fourfold increase in power generation can occur as a result of increased motor unit recruitment with some increase in skeletal muscle contractility.

Thus to explain the approximately fourfold greater power output during maximal exercise of short duration, for example during the Wingate "anaerobic" test, than during a VO_2max test, the Hill model requires that each contracting muscle fiber must be able to increase its power output fourfold. This can only be achieved with a fourfold increase in the contractility (Chapter 1) of each cross-bridge cycle.

Indeed the unpublished results from our laboratory showed that EMG activity, our measure of the extent of skeletal muscle recruitment, rose as a linear function of power output during a progressive exercise test for the measurement of VO_2max (Figure 12). But exercise terminated when EMG activity was less than about 60% of that achieved during a maximal voluntary contraction. But when subjects performed short bouts of exercise lasting between 10 and 20 seconds at progressively higher power outputs beginning at the power output at which they terminated the VO_2max test, this linear increase in EMG activity continued up to the highest power output that these subjects were able to sustain for 10-20 seconds (Figure 12).

This is not a novel finding. In his textbook [49], Enoka includes a figure (Figure 13) which also shows that only about 50% of the available motor neuron pool is activated during running whereas close to 100% of the motor neuron pool is active during a vertical jump. Thus all these findings confirm that skeletal muscle recruitment is submaximal during the VO_2max test, a finding which is completely incompatible with the A.V. Hill model.

Indeed another interesting paradox in the exercise sciences is the explanation of what constitutes "maximal" exercise. Figure 14 explains this phenomenon. The "maximal" work rate achieved during a VO_2max test in an elite cyclist might be 600W; the same athlete may be able to sustain a power output of about 2000W for a brief period during a Wingate "anaerobic" test, and perhaps an even greater power output during a vertical jump. According to the Hill model, the power output of 600W represents "maximal" exercise whereas the power output achieved during the Wingate test represents "supramaximal" exercise. But the term supramaximal is specious since by definition an exercise intensity cannot be maximal if there is another higher intensity that can also be sustained. The source of this error is the definition of the VO_2max test as a maximal test which it is not since it does not activate 100% of the available force-producing elements in the exercising limbs (Figures 10 & 12)..

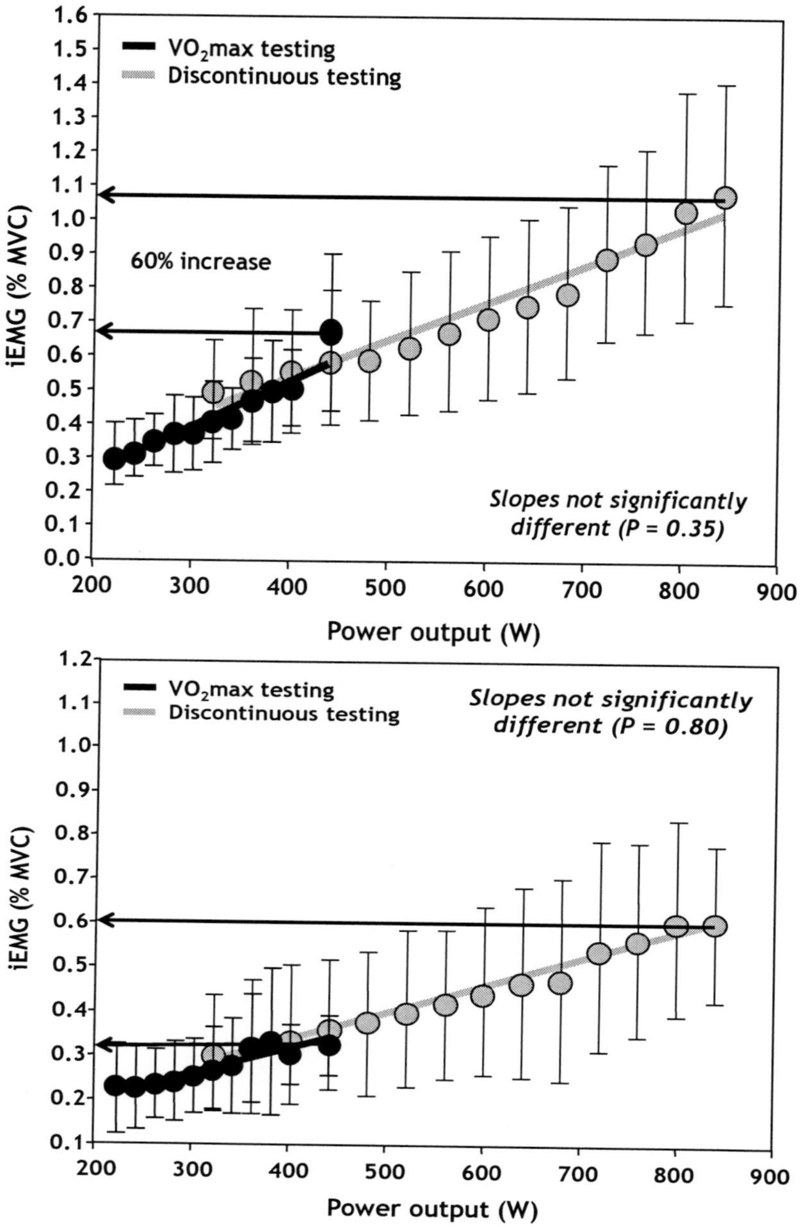

Figure 12. EMG activity (as a measure of skeletal muscle recruitment) rose as a linear function of the increasing work rate beyond that at which the VO_2max was achieved in both the Vastus Medialis (top panel) and Vastus Lateralis (bottom panel) muscles. These data confirm that skeletal muscle activation is not maximal during VO_2max testing (as is required by the Hill model).

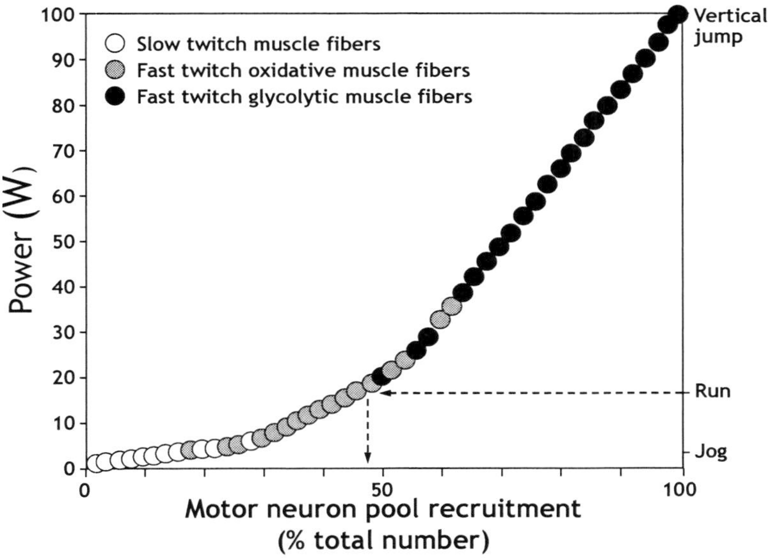

Figure 13. The textbook of Enoka [49] includes a figure showing that running requires the activation of less than about 50% of the available motor neuron pool in the exercising skeletal muscles.

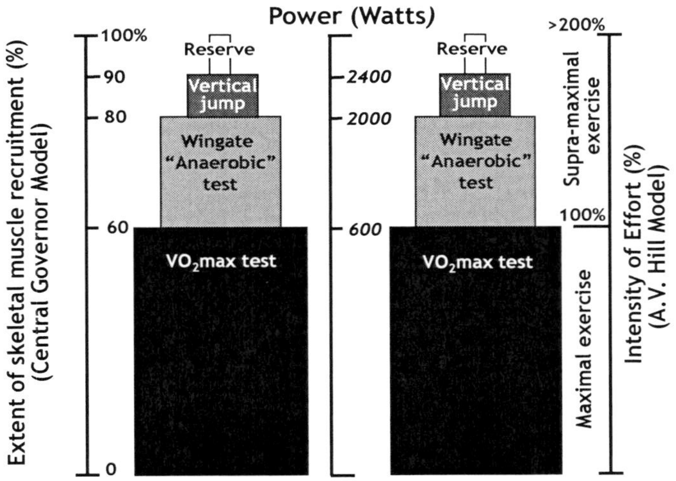

Figure 14. According to the traditional Hill model any power output (exercise intensity) greater than that at which the VO_2max is achieved, for example during the Wingate "Anaerobic" test or during a vertical jump, is "supramaximal" (right panel). But this term is specious since there is no intensity that can be higher than maximal, just as there is no state more dead than simply dead. But if all exercise intensities (power outputs) are graded according to the extent of skeletal muscle recruitment (left panel), then this specious term can be removed from the exercise science vernacular. Note that even a vertical jump does not recruit all the available motor units in the lower limbs; rather there is always some reserve capacity.

Figure 14 shows that in terms of skeletal muscle recruitment, the peak work rate of 600W achieved during the VO_2max test occurs at a submaximal level of skeletal muscle recruitment. Similarly the work rate of 2000W is achieved at a higher but still submaximal level of skeletal muscle recruitment. When these work rates are compared on a scale of the level of skeletal muscle recruitment, it is clear that both are examples of submaximal exercise.

Thus according to the CGM the intensity of any exercise bout should be related to the extent of skeletal muscle recruitment that is activated. Adopting this definition allows the specious term "supramaximal" to be removed from the accepted vernacular of our discipline.

Fifth Disproven Prediction

Fatigue does not always develop at the same level of fatiguing metabolites in the exercising limbs.

The fifth absolute requirement of the Hill model is that fatigue in any form of exercise must always develop when the concentration of metabolites causing that fatigue reach concentrations that are identical regardless of the manner in which the fatigue was produced. But there are a number of studies showing that the originally-favored fatiguing metabolite, lactic acid, is not associated with fatigue and might indeed be ergogenic. For example, the study of the Nielsen et al. [50] came to the conclusion that the accumulation of lactic acid protects against muscular fatigue so that: "In contrast to the often stated role of lactic acid as a cause of muscular fatigue, lactic acid may protect against fatigue". Many others have now come to the same conclusion [24]. In fact the unexplained paradox of the Hill model is that lactic acid needs to act selectively to impair the function of skeletal muscle whilst leaving the function of the heart and the respiratory muscles unaffected. It seems improbable that a substance that is supposedly toxic to one type of muscle can be the premier fuel for another, specifically the myocardium. This is a paradox that no one has yet challenged.

The "lactate paradox of high altitude" is perhaps the best example of an exercise condition in which exercise terminates at low blood lactate concentrations. According to one respected scientist "... the presence of the Lactate Paradox during maximal exercise at altitude is one of the strongest demonstrations of a central limitation to exercise performance"[51].

It seems more probable that the choice to either stop or to slow down during exercise is made on the basis of a complex brain decision that is influenced by a number of factors one of which might indeed be the concentration of lactate in the muscles. But it is clear that lactate does not act directly in the muscles to cause fatigue as is required by the A.V. Hill model.

Sixth Disproven Prediction

The final absolute requirement of the A.V. Hill model is that fatigue must always be absolute. Yet the reality is that athletes speed up at the end of exercise (Figure 9 in Chapter 1), the classic "endspurt", so that they cannot be absolutely fatigued. This phenomenon of the end spurt poses real problems for exercise scientists for as described in Chapter 1, it shows that our current definition of fatigue must be wrong. For the athlete's ability to speed up immediately prior to the termination of exercise proves that she was not fatigued according to the definition which holds that fatigue is present only when it is no longer possible to sustain the desired workrate. Thus according to this definition any athlete able to develop an "endspurt" is by definition not fatigued.

According to the CGM, the endspurt occurs because of an increase in skeletal muscle recruitment, perhaps associated with some increase in skeletal muscle contractility, whereas fatigue is purely an emotion [52] that is used to insure that athletes do not overexert themselves thereby threatening their homeostasis.

SUMMARY

The evidence presented here suggests that the VO_2max test is a submaximal test that terminates at less than 100% of skeletal muscle recruitment.

The protected variable that triggers the anticipatory termination of the VO_2 max test is currently unknown but may well relate to changes in blood flow to, or oxygenation of the brain [53, 54].

At high rates of respiratory ventilation, the most likely protected variable is cerebral (not myocardial or skeletal muscle) oxygenation. This is because at high rates of ventilation the carbon dioxide concentration in the blood falls and this is likely to induce cerebral vasoconstriction. This will reduce blood flow perhaps to critical parts of the brain, possibly inducing the desire to terminate the exercise.

We also propose that the exercise intensity should be defined relative to the percentage of motor units that are recruited in the exercising limbs (Figure 14). This removes the specious term "supramaximal" from the vernacular.

Finally, since the VO_2max test is "brainless", it will likely have little value in the prediction of performance in those athletic events that requires some contribution from the athlete's brain. Instead what defines the really outstanding athletes is their ability to perform a devastating end spurt. It is not clear how the VO_2max test can predict each athlete's ability to perform such an endspurt.

Thus my interpretation is that the Hill model has become a fabulous fable. It is far more likely that the brain regulates exercise performance specifically to prevent the catastrophic metabolic failure that Professor Hill and his scientific progeny believe "limits" exercise performance.

REFERENCES

[1] Taylor HL, Buskirk E, Henschel A. Maximal oxygen intake as an objective measure of cardio-respiratory performance. *J Appl Physiol*, 1955, 8, 73-80.

[2] Noakes TD, Marino FE. Arterial oxygenation, central motor output and exercise performance in humans. *J Physiol*, 2007, 585, 919-21.

[3] Noakes TD. Challenging beliefs: ex Africa semper aliquid novi: 1996 J.B. Wolffe Memorial Lecture. *Med Sci Sports Exerc*, 1997, 29, 571-90.

[4] Noakes TD. Maximal oxygen uptake: "classical" versus "contemporary" viewpoints: a rebuttal. *Med Sci Sports Exerc*, 1998, 30, 1381-98.

[5] Noakes TD, Calbet JA, Boushel R, Sondergaard H, Radegran G, Wagner PD, et al. Central regulation of skeletal muscle recruitment explains the reduced maximal cardiac output during exercise in hypoxia. *Am J Physiol Regul Integr Comp Physiol*, 2004, 287, R996-R9.

[6] Levine BD. VO2max: What do we know, and what do we still need to know? *J Physiol*, 2008, 586, 25-34.

[7] Bassett DR, Jr., Howley ET. Maximal oxygen uptake: "classical" versus "contemporary" viewpoints. *Med Sci Sports Exerc*, 1997, 29, 591-603.

[8] Bassett DR, Jr., Howley ET. Limiting factors for maximum oxygen uptake and determinants of endurance performance. *Med Sci Sports Exerc*, 2000, 32, 70-84.

[9] Bassett DR, Jr. Scientific contributions of A. V. Hill: exercise physiology pioneer. *J Appl Physiol*, 2002, 93, 1567-82.

[10] Brink-Elfegoun T, Kaijser L, Gustafsson T, Ekblom B. Maximal oxygen uptake is not limited by a central nervous system governor. *J Appl Physiol*, 2007, 102, 781-6.

[11] Hawkins MN, Snell PG, Stray-Gundersen J, Levine BD, Raven PB. Maximal oxygen uptake as a parametric measure of cardiorespiratory capacity. *Med Sci Sports Exerc*, 2007, 39, 103-7.

[12] Amann M, Romer L, Dempsey J. Reply from Markus Amann, Lee M. Romer and Jerome A. Dempsey. *J Physiol*, 2007, 585, 923-4.

[13] Shephard RJ. Is it time to retire the 'central governor'? *Sports Med*, 2009, 39, 709-21.

[14] Hopkins WG. The improbable central governor of maximal endurance performance. *Sportscience*, 2009, 13, 9-12.

[15] Brink-Elfegoun T, Holmberg HC, Ekblom MN, Ekblom B. Neuromuscular and circulatory adaptation during combined arm and leg exercise with different maximal work loads. *Eur J Appl Physiol*, 2007, 101, 603-11.

[16] Mitchell JH, Saltin B. The oxygen transport system and maximal oxygen uptake. In: Tipton CM, editor. *Exercise Physiology*: Oxford University Press; 2003; p. 255-91.

[17] Hill AV, Lupton H. Muscular exercise, lactic acid, and the supply and utilization of oxygen. *Quart J Med*, 1923, 16, 135-71.

[18] Noakes TD. How did A V Hill understand the VO2max and the "plateau phenomenon"? Still no clarity? *Br J Sports Med*, 2008, 42, 574-80.

[19] Noakes TD. Testing for maximum oxygen consumption has produced a brainless model of human exercise performance. *Br J Sports Med*, 2008, 42, 551-5.

[20] Day JR, Rossiter HB, Coats EM, Skasick A, Whipp BJ. The maximally attainable VO2 during exercise in humans: the peak vs. maximum issue. *J Appl Physiol*, 2003, 95, 1901-7.

[21] Rossiter HB, Kowalchuk JM, Whipp BJ. A test to establish maximum O2 uptake despite no plateau in the O2 uptake response to ramp incremental exercise. *J Appl Physiol*, 2006, 100, 764-70.

[22] Hill AV, Long CHN, Lupton H. Muscular exercise, lactic acid and the supply and utilisation of oxygen: parts VII-VIII. *Proc Royal Soc Bri*, 1924, 97, 155-76.

[23] Raskoff WJ, Goldman S, Cohn K. The "athletic heart". Prevalence and physiological significance of left ventricular enlargement in distance runners. *JAMA*, 1976, 236, 158-62.

[24] Noakes TD, St Clair Gibson A. Logical limitations to the "catastrophe" models of fatigue during exercise in humans. *Br J Sports Med*, 2004, 38, 648-9.

[25] Noakes TD. Physiological models to understand exercise fatigue and the adaptations that predict or enhance athletic performance. *Scand J Med Sci Sports*, 2000, 10, 123-45.

[26] Astrand PO. *Experimental studies of Physical Work Capacity in relation to sex and age* [PhD Thesis]. Copenhagen: Munksgaard; 1952.

[27] Wasserman K, Whipp BJ, Koyal SN, Beaver WL. Anaerobic threshold and respiratory gas exchange during exercise. *J Appl Physiol*, 1967, 22, 71-85.

[28] Richardson RS, Noyszewski EA, Leigh JS, Wagner PD. Lactate efflux from exercising human skeletal muscle: role of intracellular PO2. *J Appl Physiol*, 1998, 85, 627-34.

[29] Mole PA, Chung Y, Tran TK, Sailasuta N, Hurd R, Jue T. Myoglobin desaturation with exercise intensity in human gastrocnemius muscle. *Am J Physiol*, 1999, 277, R173-R80.

[30] Fletcher WM, Hopkins WG. Lactic acid in amphibian muscle. *J Physiol*, 1907, 35, 247-309.

[31] Warburton DE, Gledhill N. Counterpoint: Stroke volume does not decline during exercise at maximal effort in healthy individuals. *J Appl Physiol*, 2008, 104, 276-8.

[32] Gonzalez-Alonso J. Point: Stroke volume does/does not decline during exercise at maximal effort in healthy individuals. *J Appl Physiol*, 2008, 104, 275-6.

[33] Calbet JA, Boushel R, Radegran G, Sondergaard H, Wagner PD, Saltin B. Determinants of maximal oxygen uptake in severe acute hypoxia. *Am J Physiol Regul Integr Comp Physiol*, 2003, 284, R291-R303.

[34] Calbet JA, Boushel R, Radegran G, Sondergaard H, Wagner PD, Saltin B. Why is VO2 max after altitude acclimatization still reduced despite normalization of arterial O2 content? *Am J Physiol Regul Integr Comp Physiol*, 2003, 284, R304-R16.

[35] Calbet JA, Radegran G, Boushel R, Sondergaard H, Saltin B, Wagner PD. Effect of blood haemoglobin concentration on VO2 max and cardiovascular function in lowlanders acclimatised to 5260 m. *J Physiol*, 2002, 545, 715-28.

[36] Calbet JA, Gonzalez-Alonso J, Helge JW, Sondergaard H, Munch-Andersen T, Boushel R, et al. Cardiac output and leg and arm blood flow during incremental exercise to exhaustion on the cycle ergometer. *J Appl Physiol*, 2007, 103, 969-78.

[37] Duncker DJ, Bache RJ. Regulation of coronary blood flow during exercise. *Physiol Rev*, 2008, 88, 1009-86.

[38] Mortensen SP, Dawson EA, Yoshiga CC, Dalsgaard MK, Damsgaard R, Secher NH, et al. Limitations to systemic and locomotor limb muscle oxygen delivery and uptake during maximal exercise in humans. *J Physiol*, 2005, 566, 273-85.

[39] Noakes TD. Evidence that reduced skeletal muscle recruitment explains the lactate paradox during exercise at high altitude. *J Appl Physiol*, 2009, 106, 737-8.

[40] Wagner PD. Reduced maximal cardiac output at altitude--mechanisms and significance. *Respir Physiol*, 2000, 120, 1-11.

[41] Reeves JT, Groves BM, Sutton JR, Wagner PD, Cymerman A, Malconian MK, et al. Operation Everest II: preservation of cardiac function at extreme altitude. *J Appl Physiol*, 1987, 63, 531-9.

[42] Suarez J, Alexander JK, Houston CS. Enhanced left ventricular systolic performance at high altitude during Operation Everest II. *Am J Cardiol*, 1987, 60, 137-42.

[43] Boussuges A, Molenat F, Burnet H, Cauchy E, Gardette B, Sainty JM, et al. Operation Everest III (Comex '97): modifications of cardiac function secondary to altitude-

induced hypoxia. An echocardiographic and Doppler study. *Am J Respir Crit Care Med*, 2000, 161, 264-70.

[44] Kayser B, Narici M, Binzoni T, Grassi B, Cerretelli P. Fatigue and exhaustion in chronic hypobaric hypoxia: influence of exercising muscle mass. *J Appl Physiol*, 1994, 76, 634-40.

[45] Amann M, Eldridge MW, Lovering AT, Stickland MK, Pegelow DF, Dempsey JA. Arterial oxygenation influences central motor output and exercise performance via effects on peripheral locomotor muscle fatigue in humans. *J Physiol*, 2006, 575, 937-52.

[46] Sloniger MA, Cureton KJ, Prior BM, Evans EM. Lower extremity muscle activation during horizontal and uphill running. *J Appl Physiol*, 1997, 83, 2073-9.

[47] Sloniger MA, Cureton KJ, Prior BM, Evans EM. Anaerobic capacity and muscle activation during horizontal and uphill running. *J Appl Physiol*, 1997, 83, 262-9.

[48] Albertus Y. *Critical analysis of techniques for normalising electromyographic data* [PhD Thesis]: University of Cape Town; 2008.

[49] Enoka RM. *Neuromechanics of human movement*. Champaign, IL: Human Kinetics; 2002.

[50] Nielsen OB, de Paoli F, Overgaard K. Protective effects of lactic acid on force production in rat skeletal muscle. *J Physiol*, 2001, 536, 161-6.

[51] Brooks GA. It takes a brain. *J Appl Physiol*, 2009, 106, 743.

[52] St Clair Gibson A, Baden DA, Lambert MI, Lambert EV, Harley YX, Hampson D, et al. The conscious perception of the sensation of fatigue. *Sports Med*, 2003, 33, 167-76.

[53] Rasmussen P, Nielsen J, Overgaard M, Krogh-Madsen R, Gjedde A, Secher NH, et al. Reduced muscle activation during exercise related to brain oxygenation and metabolism in humans. *J Physiol*, 2010, 588, 1985–95.

[54] Thomas R, Stephane P. Prefrontal cortex oxygenation and neuromuscular responses to exhaustive exercise. *Eur J Appl Physiol*, 2008, 102, 153-63.

[55] Mitchell JH, Blomqvist G. Maximal oxygen uptake. *N Engl J Med*, 1971, 284, 1018-22.

In: Regulation of Fatigue in Exercise
Editor: Frank E. Marino

ISBN 978-1-61209-334-5

Chapter 6

THE ANTICIPATORY REGULATION OF FATIGUE IN EXERCISE

Frank E. Marino†
Exercise and Sports Science Laboratories & School of Human Movement Studies
Charles Sturt University, Bathurst NSW 2795, Australia

ABSTRACT

The development of fatigue during exercise has been studied for over a century and although many attempts have been made to identify the causative factors, the process by which fatigue develops is still not clearly understood. There has been much research describing the relationship between heat stress, energy availability, perception, cardiovascular perturbations, hydration, and a host of other factors impinging on the development of fatigue during exercise. Until recently it was presumed that the development of fatigue during exercise was a process moving toward system collapse. Rather, it is now clear that fatigue can also be thought of as being a process which protects the body from physiological catastrophe rather than moving toward it. In this sense it is useful to approach the understanding of fatigue by attempting to examine the potential inputs that might be used by the body to *regulate* rather than *limit* exercise performance. To this end, this chapter will explore the possible inputs which might be available to the body as a way of regulating the fatigue process and anticipating the effort required to successfully complete a given exercise task and avoid cellular catastrophe. The areas which will be discussed are the inherent differences between constant load and self-paced exercise, energy availability, thermoregulation and effort sense as possible inputs for the anticipatory regulation of fatigue in exercise.

†61 2 63384268 (Tel); †61 2 63384065 (Fax); Email: fmarino@csu.edu.au

Introduction

The ability to resist fatigue under various conditions is indeed an integral part of human performance and has been studied for well over a century. The methodological advances of scientists such as Luigi Galvani in the 1780s in experiments studying the nervous system of frogs, provided the window to further examine neuromuscular responses. In these experiments Galvani showed that frog's legs twitched in direct response to an electrical stimulus concluding at the time that the frog contained electricity [1]. However, it was the careful experimentation of scientist Alessandro Volta which showed that the frog required electrical current from another source to make the muscle twitch [1]. Through these experiments Volta had inadvertently invented the battery. Thus, the pursuit in understanding movement can be traced back to these landmark experiments which gave scientists the possibility to study the nervous system and conduct experiments which provided insights into the workings of skeletal muscle. From this time of fundamental understanding of neuromuscular response to electrical stimuli, the concept of fatigue became synonymous with the ability of the skeletal muscle to either withstand to some degree the inevitable decline in its work capacity or continue to work under given conditions.

The concept of fatigue has yielded many definitions over the centuries all of which typically place the quantitative measure of skeletal muscle force or its precipitous decrement as the major representation of fatigue. An example of a classic result which depicts the reduction in force generating capacity of the muscle is shown in Figure 1. Inevitably over the years, definitions of fatigue have emerged which attempt to more clearly define the observation depicted in Figure 1. Some of these definitions are provided in Table 1. It is clear from these definitions that the concept of fatigue has shifted to accommodate the "fine tuning" of the evolving experimental paradigms.

Table 1. Example definitions of fatigue

Author/s	Definition
Mosso (1904)	The first is the diminution of the muscular force. The second is fatigue as a sensation. That is to say, we have a physical fact which can be measured and compared, and a psychic fact which eludes measurement.
Fitts & Holloszy (1978)	A reversible state of force depression, including a lower rate of rise of force and a slower relaxation.
Bigland-Ritchie et al. (1986)	A loss of maximal force generating capacity.
Vøllestad (1997)	Any exercise-induced reduction in the maximal capacity to generate force or power output.
Allen & Westerblad (2001)	Intensive activity of muscles causes a decline in performance, known as fatigue.

References are [2, 71-74].

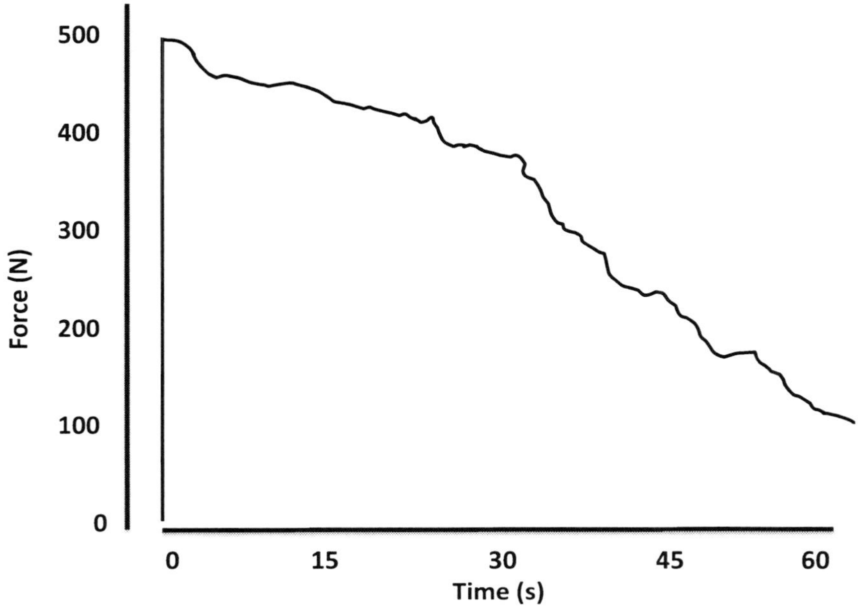

Figure 1. Shows the typical reduction in force during a sustained muscle contraction over a 60 s period when visual feedback of the force progression is available and the individual is afforded strong verbal encouragement to maintain the contraction.

Although there are many texts written on the topic of fatigue, the work produced by Mosso titled *La Fatica* (Fatigue) [2] stands as a seminal text relating the concept of fatigue to the work of the skeletal muscle. However, a much overlooked message in this text is the conclusion arrived at by Mosso after studying what he termed the "law of exhaustion" in which he categorized fatigue into two phenomena: "The first is the diminution of the muscular force. The second is fatigue as a sensation. That is to say, we have a physical fact which can be measured and compared, and a psychic fact which eludes measurement" [2](p. 154). It is interesting to note that Mosso understood that the brain played a major role in the fatigue process for he wrote "It is then not only the will, but also the nerves and the muscles which are fatigued in consequence of intense brain work" [2] (p.273). This statement reflects the development of the typical dichotomy we see today where fatigue is described as either *central* or *peripheral* in origin. This dichotomy has a particular meaning for fatigue research for it is understood that the mechanisms which cause reductions in the production of skeletal muscle force can be anywhere from the motor cortex to the skeletal muscle apparatus and all the processes which occur along this path (see chapter 4). Proponents of either the central or peripheral paradigms argue that fatigue might develop more or less in one area than the other depending on the task [3]. However, one could argue that this might not be a useful dichotomy as the human does not divide itself into discrete physiological components during exercise, rather it is a complete system which undertakes the task so that each component plays an integral part in the development of fatigue [4]. Therefore, fatigue should be viewed as a process which immediately begins upon commencing exercise rarely ending with exhaustion and seldom with irreversible physiological catastrophe [5, 6]. The evidence for this view of fatigue can be seen in studies which measure the muscle power output at various points either over time or distance. For example, when the power output was measured during a 60 min cycling time trial, the power output produced at the second time point was reduced compared to the initial value. As the total time for the exercise trial was 60 min there is no obvious or immediate reason to suspect that significant physiological changes occurred within the initial moments of exercise that would reduce the capacity of the system to produce a less than optimal effort especially if the ability to "re-produce" muscle power at the end of 60 min was similar or even higher than the initial value [7] (see Figure 2). These findings suggest that humans are able to pre-program or calculate the required effort so that the task can be completed without the system becoming exhausted. In this sense exhaustion is defined as "a total loss of strength; to consume or use up the whole of the available energy" [8].

The concept that a control system exists in which a programmer takes into consideration a finishing point (teleoanticipation) was described by Ulmer [9]. In this model, the organism would account for the various signals derived from somatosensory and metabolic changes and then make adjustments to achieve an outcome which is well within the limits of the organism's performance potential. If this system exists then it would be evident in a wide array of organisms within the animal kingdom. In fact, recent evidence indicates that this is a strategy used by migratory birds at the individual and group level if the flock is to be successful in their attempt at flying long distances [10].

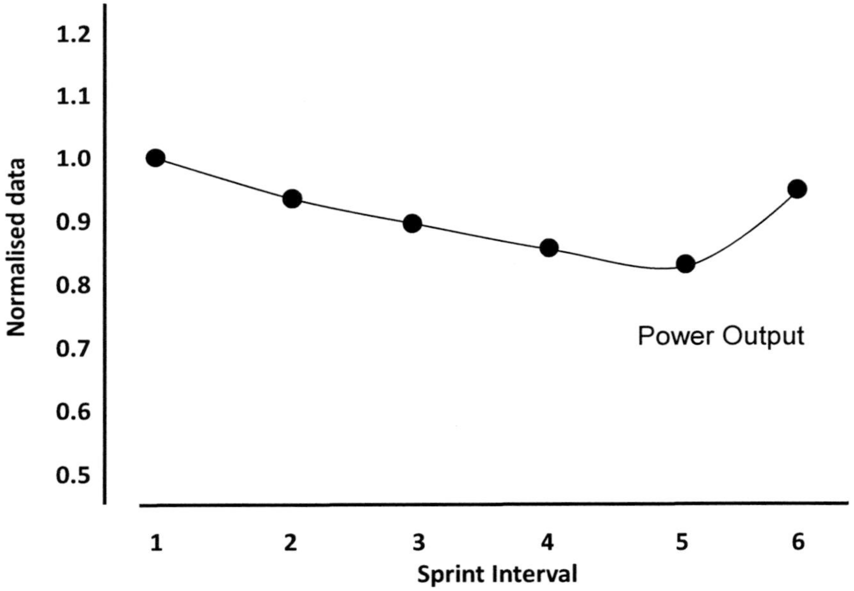

Figure 2. Shows the normalised power output during 60 min of high intensity cycling exercise. The power outputs for sprint intervals 2-6 have been normalised relative to sprint number 1. Sprint intervals occurred at each 9 min mark for a 1 min sustained effort. Note the immediate reduction in power at intervals number 2-5 compared with number 1 with an end-spurt evident at number 6 so that power output is restored to initial values. Data are re-drawn from Kay et al. [7].

The concept of fatigue during dynamic exercise requires the individual to respond on a moment-by-moment basis and it seems that there is evidence that as fatigue develops there are critical adjustments that need to be made ahead of the finishing point; the anticipatory regulation of exercise. This chapter will examine the evidence which supports such a system in nature and argue for fatigue as a process integrating many signals that develop during the course of endurance exercise allowing the organism to complete the task and avoid irreversible cellular damage.

Exercise and Laboratory Protocols

In recent times there has been debate over the appropriateness of the maximal oxygen consumption (VO_{2max}) test as a measure of the true capacity of the individual athlete [11-16]. This is not to say that this type of incremental test to exhaustion has not provided an understanding of the workings and interaction of the cardiovascular and muscular systems. Indeed the VO_{2max} test has provided a universal understanding and a point of reference from which physiologists can draw conclusions about the dynamics of human physiology. However, the inescapable principle of this test is that the subject keep pace with the experimenter or the externally driven exercise load so that voluntary termination of exercise occurs the moment a 'maximal' workload is reached where heart rate, cardiac output and stroke volume reach their maximal values so that oxygen consumption can no longer rise as originally described by Hill, Long and Lupton [17-19] and subsequently advocated by Mitcthell & Blomqvist [20]. The issue here is not whether the VO_{2max} is meaningful and ecologically valid or that it produces artifacts, rather it is the use of the resulting VO_{2max} as a reference point which is potentially problematic. That is, for the vast majority of exercise physiology experiments which examine physiological capacity, the workload is set at a percentage of the VO_{2max} (or similar outcome such as peak power output, peak velocity). Therefore, when the exercise intensity is anchored to a percentage of the 'maximum' the end result is usually time to complete the exercise. In this case exercise is completely driven by an externally imposed load rather than allowing the subject to freely adjust their intensity. In essence, the constant load model of exercise can only ever produce a result which is relative to the energy expenditure of the imposed load rather than the energy expenditure that the exercising subject is prepared or willing to "contribute" to the task. For this reason, the constant load or submaximal model of exercise can be thought of as an *open loop* task or exercise of unknown duration.

The classic result of the open loop model is depicted in Figure 3 which shows that a given treatment such as acclimation to high ambient temperature will result in relatively longer exercise time to exhaustion rather than premature fatigue in the non acclimated condition. Therefore, the consideration is whether the *open loop* model of exercise physiology reflects the true nature of the exercise response during competition or indeed the normal real-life experience of the individual. When examining this issue it is useful to consider findings which show that the reliability of the constant load model is perhaps lower than one would wish for an experimental protocol. For instance, McLellan et al. [21] have shown that time to exhaustion over a series of five trials could vary from 12 to 23.5% when exercise is set at intensities less than 80% of VO_{2max}. The authors suggested that the individual biological variation and physiological capacity might be high at lower compared with higher intensities in addition to the inherent differences between cycling and running. Interestingly, others [22] have shown that the coefficient of variation of time trial performance ranged from only 0.9 to 2.4% for highly trained and well-motivated cyclists performing four time trials over three distances. Effectively, these studies provide evidence that laboratory trials which negate the individual's ability to regulate exercise intensity did not reflect the range of physiological responses which might be present under more self regulated situations and by the level of training of the individual. It is also notable that a familiarization trial reduces the coefficient of variation significantly [23]. The issue of constant load versus self-paced exercise should not be underestimated as there are many studies which have evaluated intervention strategies attempting to overcome metabolic or thermoregulatory deficits which then advocate for particular intervention strategies based on the constant load paradigm. For example, the use of carbohydrate loading has been advocated for decades based on results of studies which show a longer exercise duration with the addition of carbohydrate to either the diet or the ingested fluid [24-28].

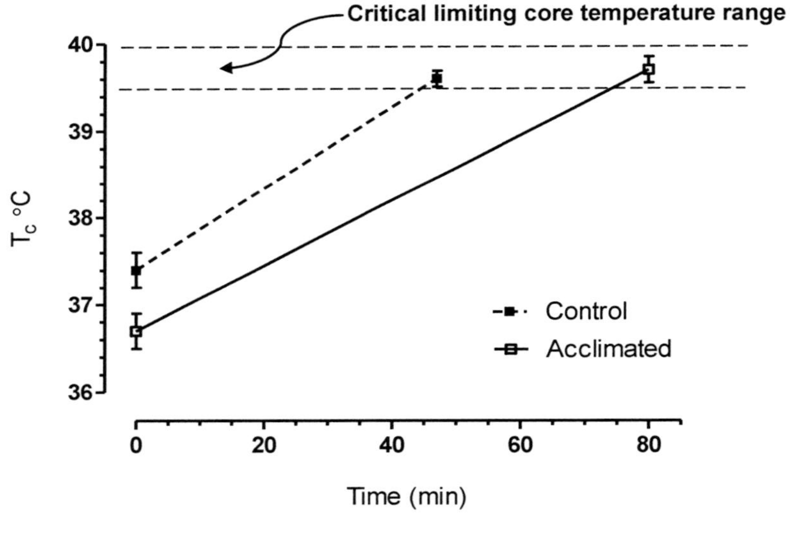

Figure 3. Shows the typical core temperature response during an *open loop* cycling exercise test when subjects were either acclimated to the heat or not (control). Note the terminal core temperature response is within a narrow range with the exercise time extended for the acclimated group (~48 min vs 80 min following acclimation). These data established the critical limiting temperature hypothesis as the common observation during open loop tests with the termination of exercise at similar core temperature irrespective of the intervention strategy. Data redrawn from Nielsen et al. [75].

Carbohydrate loading and supplementation for improved exercise performance is based largely on the findings from classic studies which used a one-legged exercise model showing that glycogen depletion in the exercised leg could be re-synthesised as much as two-fold by a 3-day carbohydrate diet [29]. Subsequently this group of researchers consistently demonstrated that carbohydrate either by feeding or infusion significantly prolonged exercise duration by sparing glycogen in the working muscle [30-33]. The classic studies of Coyle et al. [27, 28] provided differential evidence that carbohydrate feeding in the form of glucose would extend exercise duration. The findings from these and similar studies eventually led to advocating carbohydrate loading for the improvement of exercise performance in the field although they were all based on the *open loop* submaximal model of exercise physiology. However, this is not to suggest that results from these studies are of no benefit. On the contrary, the findings from these studies provide the basis on which to further explore the relationship between fuel utilisation during exercise and the fatigue process.

In contrast to the typical findings from the open loop model of exercise physiology, studies which use a self regulated exercise protocol report somewhat different findings which are not consistent with the classic view that augmented physiological responses always occur under more stressful conditions or situations which lead to a performance decrement. In the self regulated exercise model the typical scenario is that subjects either exercise for a given amount of time attempting to cover as much distance as possible or complete a given distance as quickly as possible. Therefore, if the individual commences a trial knowing either the duration or distance to be covered the protocol can be thought of as a *closed loop* model of exercise physiology. A series of studies from our laboratory using a reliable 60 min time trial punctuated with 'all out' high intensity efforts have been unable to detect any significant differences in distance covered within 60 min in either cool or in warm conditions or whether or not subjects were hyperhydrated [34-36]. Similarly, others have reported that a carbohydrate diet which increased muscle glycogen concentrations did not result in improved performance in a 100 km time trial [37]. Therefore, in self regulated exercise where subjects are required to cover a distance as quickly as possible the physiological response is regulated in such a way that the distance to be covered is achieved and premature termination of exercise seldom ensues. This outcome contrasts the constant load model which predicts reduced exercise duration under stressful conditions rather than the resulting longer duration of the self-paced trial.

EVIDENCE FOR ANTICIPATORY REGULATION

The classic understanding is that exercise capacity is governed by systemic and cellular limitations that when achieved lead to catastrophic cellular events thereby limiting physical exertion; the so-called catastrophe model [38]. This physiological paradigm gained acceptance as it was thought that the heart limited the availability of oxygen to the working muscle leading to anaerobiosis and eventually to the cessation of exercise [17, 39]. This view has been challenged on the basis that the availability of oxygen to the heart is also limiting leading to myocardial ischemia, but since ischemia does not occur during exercise in health this physiological model is limited in its predictability [13, 40]. This debate is beyond the scope of the present discussion so the interested reader should consult the relevant readings (see chapters 1 & 5). Regardless of one's point of view on the putative cause limiting exercise performance, it is an unavoidable conclusion that sporting events require the individual to give an effort which will sustain them well beyond the end of the event. On this basis alone it is likely that during a sporting event requiring sustained effort, individuals likely plan a strategy ahead of time which will take into account the amount of energy required to complete the task. This understanding is not particularly new as many athletes recognise this as *pacing*. A prime example of pacing was the record-breaking mile run by Sir Roger Bannister in 1954. In his recording of that historic event, Roger Bannister described the moments in the race where his friends and fellow runners Chris Brasher and Chris Chataway undertook a pacing strategy leading to success: "We seemed to be going slowly! Impatiently I shouted 'Faster!' But Brasher kept his head and did not change the pace. I went on worrying until I heard the first lap time, 57.5 seconds. In the excitement my knowledge of pace had deserted me. Brasher could have run the first quarter in 55 seconds without my realising it, because I felt so full of running, but I should have had to pay for it later. Instead, he had made success possible" [41](p.165). Although anecdotal, this description of the events of 1954 does make the point that there must be an individual strategy to success in sporting events.

However, anecdotal evidence from sporting events does not necessarily constitute reliable evidence for anticipatory regulation of exercise performance. Experimental evidence for anticipatory regulation comes from the studies of Williamson et al. [42] where subjects cycled at a constant load for 15 min on three separate occasions after being hypnotised to respond to either uphill, downhill, or level gradient. These authors found that the mere suggestion of an uphill gradient increased the heart rate response significantly above that of the level gradient even though under all three conditions the gradient was actually identical. However, the heart rate response during the downhill gradient was not different from that achieved during the level gradient. Interestingly, the rating of perceived exertion (RPE) was increased significantly when subjects were told they were cycling uphill compared to the level gradient. Furthermore, the RPE decreased when subjects believed they were cycling downhill. These findings indicate that physiological responses might be related to an expectation in addition to the actual work that needed to be undertaken, for there seems to be a minimum cardiovascular response to the exercise to sustain a given metabolic demand. However, these authors also measured regional cerebral blood flow (rCBF) distribution during the three different hypnotic exercise tests and found that this particular variable changed according to whether there was a suggestion of downhill cycling or uphill cycling. For instance, the suggestion of downhill cycling produced a decrease in rCBF in a region of the anterior cingulate cortex and the left insular cortex. Others have shown that activation of the anterior cingulate cortex is closely related to a perceived change in unpleasantness of painful stimuli [43]. Therefore, the reduction in RPE with the suggestion of downhill cycling might indicate that specific brain regions are related to the interpretation of unpleasantness and are activated not solely by the actual physical effort but the perceived effort. Conversely, with the suggestion of uphill cycling there were increases in rCBF to the right thalamic region and the insular cortex. Although involved in regulation of many cardiovascular and respiratory responses, the insular cortex is also thought to serve as a site for 'central command' activating motor areas by feedforward signals [44]. Even given the limitations which exist with respect to hypnotic manipulation such as hemisphere dominance; based on these particular data it is entirely reasonable to suggest that there exist both brain regions and pathways which would allow for the anticipatory or feedforward regulation of the expected exercise.

Perhaps the strongest evidence for the feedforward regulation of exercise comes from studies which manipulate heat strain under various conditions. The interpretation of data from thermoregulatory studies is very dependent on assumptions that the body or indeed the brain has limited tolerance to the amount of heat it can store [45]. For instance, it has been widely thought that there exists a critical limiting core temperature which is associated with a reduction in motor drive leading to premature fatigue (see also Figure 3) [46-48]. However, recent field studies have provided evidence that a critical limiting core temperature may be an artifact observed in typical laboratory settings [49, 50]. When comparing African with Caucasian runners in elevated ambient temperatures, it was found that the African runners were able to maintain higher running speeds whilst the Caucasian runners decreased their running speed even though core temperature was identical at the commencement of the performance run [51]. This particular finding could only be explained on the basis that the heavier Caucasian runners had to reduce their pace and thereby reduce their heat retention to avoid a lethal hyperpyrexia. However, this reduction in pace could only occur by forecasting the thermal limits as the point of fatigue would be too late to reduce the motor drive to avoid thermal injury. This view was subsequently confirmed by Tucker et al. [52] who showed that during a 20 km self-paced cycle time trial under cool and hot conditions, subjects reduced their power output and integrated electromyographic (iEMG%) signal in the heat well before there was a significant difference in rectal temperature and which only occurred at the end of the time trial. These authors proposed "... that the early decline in power output in the absence of any thermoregulatory disturbance in the heat forms part of an anticipatory response in the brain, which mediates a reduction in skeletal muscle recruitment to ensure that the rate of heat production is reduced" (p. 428).

Notably, in an attempt to disapprove the existence of an anticipatory mechanism operating during exercise and heat stress Ely et al. [49] investigated the heat storage response over 8 km on a circular running track so that split times were recorded every 200 m. A notable finding in this study was that 12 of the 24 runners exceeded a rectal temperature of 40°C during the trial. A rectal temperature greater than 40°C was not associated with a reduction in performance in the 8 km time trial and runners were actually able to accelerate in the final 600 m despite having a rectal temperature above 39.5°C. The authors concluded that pace is independent of the heat storage in both warm and cool conditions as runners appeared to be able to accelerate despite the high rate of heat storage, so an anticipatory reduction in pace was unlikely. This conclusion negates the fact that participants commenced the trial in warm conditions at a velocity of about 295 m/min and then within 600 m had reduced their running velocity to just under 280 m/min. The velocity was further reduced in the last 50% of the time trial to under 280 m/min only to return to a pace above 280 m/min within the final 200 m of the trial. In comparison, the running velocity in the cooler condition was maintained throughout the trial but with an end-spurt again evident in the final stages. It is an unavoidable conclusion that a change in pace no matter how small is mediated by changes in muscle recruitment and by extension a change in the heat generating capacity of the muscle.

The extent to which motor drive is regulated under different levels of inspired oxygen has been studied by Amann et al. [53, 54]. In these studies, participants were required to cycle 5 km in the fastest time possible while exposed to either room air (normoxia, FIO_2 0.21), hypoxia ($F\ IO_2$ 0.15), iso-oxia ($F\ IO_2$ 0.24-0.30) or hyperoxia ($F\ IO_2$ 1.0). Under these conditions there was increased arterial oxygen content from hypoxia to hyperoxia resulting in parallel increases in central neural output (43%), power output (30%) and improved time trial performance (12%). It was also evident that from hyperoxia to normoxia there was an immediate reduction in power output and EMG response approaching each 1 km distance only for these variables to return to near initial values at the completion of the trial. The authors suggested that the effect of arterial oxygen content "is a significant determinant of the magnitude of central motor output during exercise in order to prevent 'excessive' development of peripheral muscle fatigue beyond a critical threshold or sensory tolerance limit" [53][p. 950]. However, a different interpretation of these findings has been posited suggesting that an 'endspurt' in which power output and EMG activity increase at the end of exercise when F IO_2 values are 1.0 and 0.28, disproves the conclusion that central motor output is regulated principally by feedback from the fatiguing skeletal muscles. That is, a system which responds only to sensory feedback could not permit an 'endspurt' as it could not forecast the extent of the fatigue at the finish of the 'endspurt'. As suggested by Tucker et al. [55], when participants performed two 20 km cycling time trials in either hyperoxia or normoxia, improved exercise performance in the hyperoxia trial was due to the maintenance of a higher power output throughout the trial and a higher iEMG% at various points. Again, in this study an endspurt was evident in both hyperoxia and the normoxia trials so that peak values were observed at the conclusion of the 20 km. Therefore, changes in muscle recruitment and work rate seem to be dependent and sensitive to the oxygen content of inspired air. The fact that higher power outputs and muscle recruitment were maintained with higher oxygen content in the inspired air whilst these variables were reduced almost immediately after the commencement of exercise only to return to near peak values at the end of exercise, indicates that pacing strategies and performance are the result of feedforward, anticipatory adjustments in power output.

More recent studies have examined the adjustment of performance and motor output relative to the availability of supplemental energy. The intravenous infusion of glucose which provides carbohydrate in the circulation had no effect on the time to complete a 60 min cycle time trial compared with the infusion of saline placebo [56]. Conversely, the regular rinsing of the mouth with a non-sweet moltodextrin solution which was highly unlikely to have any direct effect on circulating glucose levels did reduce the time to complete a performance trial [57]. The conclusion from these studies was that there exist taste receptors in the mouth which are both sensitive to non-sweet carbohydrates and influence neural pathways which improve exercise performance. Subsequent to these studies Chambers et al. [58] evaluated the effect of mouth rinsing with solutions containing glucose and moltodextrin disguised with artificial sweetner (placebo) on cycle time trial performance. In both carbohydrate and moltodextrin trials the total work was completed in faster time compared with the placebo. It was also shown that the functional magnetic resonance imaging (*f*MRI) studies identified brain regions which were activated by both carbohydrate and moltodextrin solutions whilst artificial sweetners had no such effect. These authors suggested that improvement in performance was mediated by the presence of carbohydrate in the mouth by activating the brain regions thought to be related to reward and motor control. More recent work shows that following fatiguing contractions, rinsing the mouth with carbohydrate modifies corticomotor excitability and voluntary force production so there is immediate ergogenic effects which precede any substrate or endocrine signalling associated with the ingestion [59]. These findings provide evidence for the existence of a neural pathway integrating sensorimotor signals permitting immediate recruitment of both fatigued and fresh muscle in anticipation of receiving the substrate for utilization at the contraction site. Thus, it is now apparent, at least for energy consumption purposes, that there are neural networks which give rise to an anticipatory or feedforward mechanism signalling the availability of energy.

The feedforward regulation of energy availability and utilisation for the purpose of continuing exercise provides a novel approach to understanding the fatigue process. For example, following a CHO loading trial Rauch et al. [60] found that mean power output and muscle glycogen utilisation was higher during a 60 min cycle time trial compared to when subjects consumed their normal diet. Remarkably, although the CHO loading trial resulted in a higher mean power output and faster time trial performance (36.55 vs 38.1 km/h), the end of exercise muscle glycogen content was similar (18 vs 20 mmol/kg w/w). There are two significant conclusions that can be drawn from these findings. First, the similar end of exercise muscle glycogen concentration despite the difference in the pre-exercise concentration is indicative of a pacing strategy which is 'constrained' by a 'critical' level of substrate availability. Second, because subjects decreased their power outputs over the initial 30-32 min of the 60 min trial when muscle glycogen concentrations were relatively high, but were then able to increase their power outputs in the last 2 min of the trial when muscle glycogen was perhaps at the lowest value, indicates that muscle power output was reduced for the first 58 min of the 60 min time trial by an anticipatory pacing strategy. These results do not support the classical understanding which posits that critically low levels of muscle glycogen concentrations lead to metabolite induced fatigue due to an inability to rapidly generate ATP from glycolytic pathways. For if this was true, it would not be possible to generate the greatest power output after 58 min when substrate availability was at its lowest.

The Sense of Effort and Anticipatory Regulation

The emotional state of the individual has attracted much research in an effort to understand the relationship between the physical and mental responses for any given set of circumstances. In fact, Charles Darwin provided a treatise on the expressions of emotions in both man and animals in an attempt to describe the role of the brain in such responses [61]. Since this landmark writing other theories describing the emotions of humans have been developed including the classical James-Lang Theory and the Cannon-Bard Theory [62, 63] which argue for a direct relationship between the physical and emotional response. There are also documented accounts of people surviving extreme situations based largely on the ability to 'conjure assistance from the mind' [64]. However, advances in neuroscience methodologies such as brain imaging have provided novel insights into conscious and unconscious emotions [65]. Therefore, it is not only useful to consider the emotional state during exercise but it is also impossible to completely separate it from the physical or physiological response.

Borg [66] has written that "of all single indicators of the degree of physical strain, perceived exertion is one of the most informative" (p. 560) and therefore has become one of the often utilised tools to measure the subjective response to the difficulty of the exercise. In this sense it is useful to view the rating of perceived exertion (RPE) as an integration of signals given its positive correlation with heart rate, power output, oxygen uptake, blood lactate and respiratory rate [67]. The question to be addressed, therefore, is how the RPE provides for anticipatory regulation of exercise.

There are now several studies and re-interpretations of existing data which strongly suggest that RPE is a critical signal for an anticipatory response. When participants performed constant load exercise to volitional fatigue in either a glycogen-loaded or glycogen-depleted state, the exercise time was determined by the rate of increase in RPE [68]. The salient point from these findings is that the initial and the end of exercise RPE were similar for both conditions even though the rate of rise in RPE was higher for the glycogen-depleted condition. However, when the RPE was expressed relative to the time taken to complete the exercise, the RPE increased in a linear fashion for both conditions. These finding indicate that RPE is perhaps determined by the state of energy availability given that the rate of increase in RPE was higher for the glycogen-depleted condition. The other important interpretation relates to the fact that the RPE increased at different rates for both conditions from the start of exercise. This indicates that the perception of effort is inextricably linked to energy availability so that energy expenditure will not exceed that which would otherwise lead to physiological catastrophe. That is, RPE was possibly set in anticipation to ensure that the maximal RPE was achieved well before substrate availability was depleted.

Similarly, when subjects were required to 'clamp' their RPE [16/20] whilst cycling in either 15, 25 or 35°C (65% relative humidity) environments, the reductions in power output were linear in all trials but the rate of decline was greatest in 35°C [69]. However, the decline in power output occurred well ahead of any differences in rectal temperature between trials. This result indicates that subjects adjusted their power output in anticipation of the rise in rectal temperature by altering the number of active motor units as evidenced by the reduction in integrated EMG during the 35°C trial. Remarkably, the EMG was then increased well above the initial value at the end of the trial. Therefore, changes in work rate and hence, motor unit recruitment, were achieved specifically to maintain the RPE at the predetermined level, suggesting that afferent feedback, effort sense and work rate are co-dependent.

A further and interesting observation is that when administered a dopamine/ noreadrenaline re-uptake inhibitor; compared to a placebo, participants were able to complete a time trial performance in the heat (30°C) significantly faster (~36.4 min vs ~39.8 min) and with a significantly higher terminal rectal temperature (40°C vs 39.7°C) [70]. However, the faster time trial in the heat was accomplished with an identical RPE to that achieved in the placebo trial. This suggests that effort sense manifested as the RPE was 'mismatched' or possibly even 'up-regulated' due to the action of the drug, allowing more work to be performed as a consequence of altered arousal and motivation.

CONCLUSION

Anticipatory regulation of exercise is a relatively new school of thought in the exercise and sports sciences. However, athletes recognize this as pacing and although a pacing strategy is not a new concept there is no definitive mechanism identified by which a pacing strategy is developed other than to assume that previous experience plays a role. Much of the current evidence is based on the changes in work rate or power output over time and the changes in motor unit recruitment and de-recruitment during exercise. The inputs which determine the changes in the recruitment pattern of motor units during exercise are most likely a key component. The inputs which permit anticipatory regulation of exercise might include energy availability, rate of heat storage, oxygen availability and sensing and as yet undiscovered inputs from other sources. The possibility that there exists a mechanism for anticipatory regulation of exercise provides an enticing avenue in the study of fatigue and the understanding of performance regulation.

REFERENCES

[1] Dougan A. *Raising the dead: the men who created Frankenstein.* Edinburgh: Birlinn Limited; 2008.

[2] Mosso A. *Fatigue.* London: Swan Sonnenschein & Co. Ltd; 1904.

[3] Schillings M, Hoefsloot W, Stegeman D, Zwarts M. Relative contributions of central and peripheral factors to fatigue during a maximal sustained effort. *Eur J Appl Physiol.* 2003, 90, 562-8.

[4] Marino FE, Gard M, Drinkwater E. The limits to exercise performance and the future of fatigue research *Br J Sports Med.* 2011, 45, 65-67.

[5] Noakes TD, St Clair Gibson A. Logical limitations to the "catastrophe" models of fatigue during exercise in humans. *Br J Sports Med.* 2004, 38, 648-9.

[6] Lambert EV, St Clair Gibson A, Noakes TD. Complex systems model of fatigue: integrative homeostatic control of peripheral physiological systems during exercise in humans. *Br J Sports Med.* 2005, 39, 52-62.

[7] Kay D, Marino FE, Cannon J, St Clair Gibson A, Lambert MI, Noakes TD. Evidence for neuromusclur fatigue during high-intensity cycling in warm, humid conditions. *Eur J Appl Physiol.* 2001, 84, 115-21.

[8] *The Australian concise Oxford dictionary.* 4th ed. South Melbourne: Oxford University Press; 2004.

[9] Ulmer HV. Concept of extracellular regulation of muscular metabolic rate during heavy exercise in humans by psychophysiological feedback. *Experentia.* 1996, 52, 416-20.

[10] Nagy M, Ákos Z, Biro D, Vicsek T. Hierarchical group dynamics in pigeon flocks. *Nature.* 2010, 464, 890-3.

[11] Noakes TD. Maimal oxygen uptke: "classical" versus "contemporary" viewpoints: a rebuttal. *Med Sci Sports Exerc.* 1998, 9, 1381-98.

[12] Noakes TD. Maximal oxygen uptake as a parametric measure of cardiorespiratory capacity: Comment. *Med Sci Sports Exerc.* 2008, 40, 585.

[13] Noakes TD. Testing for maximum oxygen consumption has produced a brainless model of human exercise performance. *Br J Sports Med.* 2008, 42, 551-5.

[14] Noakes TD, Marino FE. Point/Counterpoint: Maximal oxygen uptake is limited by a central nervous system governor. *J Appl Physiol.* 2008, 106, 338-48.

[15] Bassett DRJ, Howley ET. Maximal oxygen uptake: "classical" versus "contemporary" viewpoints. *Med Sci Sports Exerc.* 1997, 29, 591-603.

[16] Bassett DRJ, Howley ET. Limiting factors for maximum oxygen uptake and determinants of endurance performance. *Med Sci Sports Exerc.* 2000, 32, 70-84.

[17] Hill AV, Long CHN, Lupton H. Muscular exercise, lactic acid and the supply and utilisation of oxygen : parts VII-VIII. *Proceedings of the Royal Society of Britain.* 1924, 97, 155-76.

[18] Hill AV, Long CHN, Lupton H. Muscular exercise, lactic acid, and the supply utilization of oxygen:Parts I-III. *Proceedings of the Royal Society of Britain.* 1924, 96, 438-75.

[19] Hill AV, Lupton H. Muscular exercise, lactic acid, and the supply and utilization of oxygen. *Q J Med.* 1923, 16, 135-71.

[20] Mitchell J, Blomqvist G. Maximal oxygen uptake. *N Engl J Med.* 1971, 284, 1018.

[21] McLellan TM, Cheung SS, Jacobs I. Variability of time to exhaustion during submaximal exercise. *Can J Appl Physiol.* 1995, 20, 39-51.

[22] Hickey MS, Costill DL, McConell GK, Widrick JJ, Tanaka H. Day to day variation in time trial cycling performance *Int J Sports Med.* 1992, 13, 467-70.

[23] Marino FF, Kay D, Serwach N, Hilder M, Preston P. A reproducible and variable intensity cycling performance protocol for warm humid conditions. *J Sci Med Sport.* 2002, 5, 95-107.

[24] Below PR, Mora- Rodriguez R, Gonzalez-Alonso J, Cotle EF. Fluid and carbohydrate ingestion independently improve performance during 1 h of intense exercise. *Med Sci Sports Exerc.* 1995, 27, 200-10.

[25] Burke LM. Nutritional needs for exercise in the heat. *Comp Biochem Physiol.* 2001, 128, 735-48.

[26] Coggan AR, Coyle EF. Reversal of fatigue during prolonged exercise by carbohydrate infusion or ingestion. *J Appl Physiol.* 1987, 63, 23888-2395.

[27] Coyle E, Hagberg J, Hurley B, Martin W, Ehsani A, Holloszy J. Carbohydrate feeding during prolonged strenuous exercise can delay fatigue. *J Appl Physiol.* 1983, 55, 230-5.

[28] Coyle EF, Coggan AR, Hemmert MK, Ivy JL. Muscle glycogen utilization during prolonged strenuous exercise when fed carbohydrate. *J Appl Physiol.* 1986, 61, 165-72.

[29] Bergström J, Hultman E. Muscle glycogen synthesis after exercise: an enhancing factor localized to the muscle cells in man. *Nature.* 1966, 210, 309-10.

[30] Bergström J, Hermansen L, Hultman E, Saltin B. Diet, muscle glycogen and physical performance. *Acta Physiol Scand.* 1967, 71, 140-50.

[31] Bergström J, Hultman E. A study of the glycogen metabolism during exercise in man. *Scand J Clin Lab Invest.* 1967, 19, 218-28.

[32] Hermansen L, Hultman E, Saltin B. Muscle glycogen during prolonged severe exercise. *Acta Physiol Scand.* 1967, 71, 129-39.

[33] Hultman E. Muscle glycogen in man determined in needle biopsy specimens method and normal values. *Scand J Clin Lab Invest.* 1967, 19, 209-17.

[34] Kay D, Marino FE. Failure of fluid ingestion to improve self-paced exercise performance in moderate-to-warm humid environments. *J Therm Biol.* 2003, 28, 29-34.

[35] Marino FE, Cannon J, Kay D. Neuromuscular responses to hydration in moderate to warm ambient conditions during self-paced high intensity exercise. *Br J Sports Med.* 2010, 44, 961-967.

[36] Marino FE, Kay D, Cannon J. Glycerol hyperhydration fails to improve endurance performance and thermoregulation in humans in a warm humid environment. *Pflügers Archives.* 2003, 446, 445-62.

[37] Burke LM, Hawley JA, Schabort EJ, St Clair Gibson A, Mujika I, Noakes TD. Carbohydrate loading failed to improve 100-km cycling performance in a placebo trial. *J Appl Physiol.* 2000, 88, 1284-90.

[38] Edwards RHT. Biochemical bases of fatigue in exercise performance: catastrophe theory of muscular fatigue. In: Knuttgen HG, Vogel JA, Poortmans J, editors. *Biochemistry of exercise. Champagne, Il: Human Kinetics Publishers;* 1983. p. 3 - 27.

[39] Noakes TD. Physiological models to understand exercise fatigue and the adaptations that predict or enhance athletic performance. *Scand J Med Sci Sports.* 2000, 10, 123-45.

[40] Noakes TD. How did AV Hill understand the VO2max and the "plateau phenomenon"? Still no clarity? *Br J Sports Med.* 2008;42:574.
[41] Bannister R. *The first four minutes.* Phoenix Mill, UK: Sutton Publishing; 2004.
[42] Williamson JW, McColl R, Mathews D, Mitchell JH, Raven PB, Morgan WP. Hypnotic manipulation of effort sense during dynamic exercise: cardiovascular responses and brain activation. *J Appl Physiol.* 2001, 90, 1392-9.
[43] Rainville P, Duncan G, Price D, Carrier B, Bushnell M. Pain affect encoded in human anterior cingulate but not somatosensory cortex. *Sci.* 1997, 277, 968.
[44] Waldrop T, Eldridge F, Iwamoto G, Mitchell J. Central neural control of respiration and circulation during exercise. *Handbook of Physiology Exercise: Regulation and Integration of Multiple Systems.* 1996, 333-80.
[45] Gisolfi CV, Mora F. *The hot brain: survival, temperature and the human body. Massachusetts:* MIT Press; 2000.
[46] González-Alonso J, Teller C, Anderson SL, Jensen FB, Hyldig T, Nielsen B. Influence of body temperature on the development of fatigue during prolonged exercise in the heat. *J Appl Physiol.* 1999, 86, 1032-9.
[47] Walters TJ, Ryan KL, Tate LM, Mason PA. Exercise in the heat is limited by a critical internal temperature. *J Appl Physiol.* 2000, 89, 799-806.
[48] Nybo L, Nielsen B. Hyperthermia and central fatigue during prolonged exercise in humans. *J Appl Physiol.* 2001, 91, 1055-60.
[49] Ely BR, Ely MR, Cheuvront SN, Kenefick RW, DeGroot DW, Montain SJ. Evidence against a 40 °C core temperature threshold for fatigue in humans. *J Appl Physiol.* 2009, 107, 1519-25.
[50] Byrne C, Lee JKW, Chew SAN, Lim CL, Tan EYM. Continuous thermoregulatory responses to mass-participation distance running in heat. *Med Sci Sports Exerc.* 2006, 38, 803-10.
[51] Marino FE, Lambert MI, Noakes TD. Superior performance of African runners in warm humid but not in cool environmental conditions. *J Appl Physiol.* 2004, 96, 124-30.
[52] Tucker R, Rauch L, Harley YXR, Noakes TD. Impaired exercise performance in the heat associated with an anticipatory reduction in skeletal muscle recruitment. *Pflügers Archives.* 2004, 448, 422-30.
[53] Amann M, Eldridge MW, Lovering AT, Stickland MK, Pegelow DF, Dempsey JA. Arterial oxygenation influences central motor output and exercise performance via effects on peripheral locomotor muscle fatigue in humans. *J Physiol.* 2006, 575, 937-52.
[54] Amann M, Romer LM, Subudhi AW, Pegelow DF, Dempsey JA. Severity of arterial hypoxaemia affects the relative contributions of peripheral muscle fatigue to exercise performance in healthy humans. *J Physiol.* 2007, 581, 389-403.
[55] Tucker R, Kayser B, Rae E, Rauch L, Bosch A, Noakes T. Hyperoxia improves 20 km cycling time trial performance by increasing muscle activation levels while perceived exertion stays the same. *Eur J Appl Physiol.* 2007, 101, 771-81.
[56] Carter JM, Jeukendrup AE, Mann CH, Jones DA. The effect of glucose infusion on glucose kinetics during 1-h time trial. *Med Sci Sports Exerc.* 2004, 36, 1543-50.
[57] Carter JM, Jeukendrup AE, Jones DA. The effect of carbohydrate mouth rinse on 1-h cycle time trial performance. *Med Sci Sports Exerc.* 2004, 36, 2107-11.

[58] Chambers E, Bridge M, Jones D. Carbohydrate sensing in the human mouth: effects on exercise performance and brain activity. *J Physiol.* 2009, 587, 1779-94.

[59] Gant N, Stinear C, Byblow W. Carbohydrate in the mouth immediately facilitates motor output. *Brain Res.* 2010, 1350, 151-158.

[60] Rauch HGL, St Clair Gibson A, Lambert EV, Noakes TD. A signalling role for muscle glycogen in the regulation of pace during prolonged exercise. *Br J Sports Med.* 2005, 39, 34-8.

[61] Darwin CR. *The expression of the emotions in man and animals.* London: John Murray; 1872.

[62] James W. *What is an emotion? Mind.* 1884, 9, 188-205.

[63] Cannon WB. The James-Lang theory of emotion. *Am J Psychol.* 1927, 39, 106-24.

[64] Geiger J. *The third man factor: the secret to suvival in extreme environments.* Melbourne, Australia: Text Publishing Company; 2009.

[65] Dolan R. Emotion, cognition, and behavior. *Science.* 2002, 298, 1191.

[66] Borg G. Psychophysical scaling with applications in physical work and the perception of exertion. *Scand J Work Environ Health.* 1990, 16, 55-8.

[67] Robertson R. Central signals of perceived exertion during dynamic exercise. *Med Sci Sports Exerc.* 1982, 14, 390-6.

[68] Noakes TD, Snow RJ, Febbraio MA. Linear relationship between the perception of effort and the duration of constant load exercise that remains. *J Appl Physiol.* 2004, 96, 1571-3.

[69] Tucker R, Marle T, Lambert EV, Noakes TD. The rate of heat storage mediates an anticipatory reduction in exercise intensity during cycling at a fixed rating of perceived exertion. *J Physiol.* 2006, 574, 905-15.

[70] Watson P, Hasegawa H, Roelands B, Piacentini MF, Looverie R, Meeusen R. Acute dopamine/noradrenaline reuptake inhibition enhances human exercise performance in warm, but not temperate conditions. *J Physiol.* 2005, 565, 873-83.

[71] Fitts R, Holloszy J. Effects of fatigue and recovery on contractile properties of frog muscle. *J Appl Physiol.* 1978, 45, 899.

[72] Bigland-Ritchie B, Furbush F, Woods JJ. Fatigue of intermittent submaximal voluntary contractions: central and peripheral factors. *J Appl Physiol.* 1986, 61, 421-9.

[73] Vøllestad N. Measurement of human muscle fatigue. *J Neurosci Methods.* 1997, 74, 219-27.

[74] Allen D, Westerblad H. Role of phosphate and calcium stores in muscle fatigue. *J Physiol.* 2001, 536, 657.

[75] Nielsen B, Hales JRS, Strange S, Christensen NJ, Warberg J, Saltin B. Human circulatory and thermoregulatory adaptations with heat acclimation and exercise in a hot, dry environment. *J Physiol.* 1993, 460, 467-85.

In: Regulation of Fatigue in Exercise
Editor: Frank E. Marino

ISBN 978-1-61209-334-5

Chapter 7

FATIGUE AND THE REGULATION OF EXERCISE INTENSITY DURING TEAM SPORT MATCHES

Rob Duffield[1,*] and Aaron J. Coutts[2]
[1] School of Human Movement Studies, Charles Sturt University
Panorama Ave, Bathurst, NSW2795, Australia
[2] School of Leisure, Sport and Tourism, University of Technology, Sydney
Kuring-gai Campus, NSW 2070, Australia

ABSTRACT

Despite the engaging discussion concerning the mechanisms of fatigue during exercise, one common theme seems apparent; that the underlying mechanisms are intensity and duration dependent. As expected, the debate regarding the definition, presence and mechanisms of exercise-induced fatigue centres heavily on findings of laboratory investigations. However, presently there is little evidence from ecologically valid, field-based settings to support this laboratory evidence. From the view of the Exercise and Sports Sciences, a central tenant of the research into the mechanisms of fatigue is to transfer the findings back to an applied setting to understand exercise performance in the field. Accordingly, many laboratory studies have investigated mechanisms responsible for the amelioration or termination of exercise performance. However, particularly for team sports, the poor ecological validity of exercise protocols used restricts application of the findings to the field. Further, termination of exercise in the field is normally associated with the end of a game, rather than volitional exhaustion, reducing the application of laboratory findings to competition settings. Recently, the use of player tracking technology has increased the ease and resolution of collecting game-based data to understand movement patterns of team sport athletes. As such, from the growing body of literature it is possible to gain insight into the regulation of game-based exercise intensity and hence postulate as to the mechanisms responsible for the fluctuations in exercise patterns. Added to these findings are further game-based data of

* +61 2 6338 4939 (Tel); +61 2 6338 4065 (Fax); E-mail: rduffield@csu.edu.au

physiological responses and the effects of changing conditions on the resulting exercise patterns. Accordingly, from a collection of game-based data for a range of team sports, it is possible to develop a more ecologically valid description of the influence of transient and absolute fatigue, or more aptly, the regulation of exercise intensity. This chapter will discuss game-based data on the motion characteristics of players, along with a range of physiological data collected from 'real-world' settings. To supplement this, using hot environmental conditions as an example, further analysis of how changing environments affect the regulation of exercise patterns will also be addressed. Finally, from these respective collections of data, the role and influence of potential mechanisms highlighted by laboratory evidence will be discussed. As such, this chapter will examine the patterns of exercise regulation and postulate on the possible underlying mechanisms responsible for fatigue during team sport exercise.

INTRODUCTION

Fatigue is defined as the inability to maintain the required or imposed work rate [1]. In recent times, the term 'fatigue' has been used to refer to both the transient reduction in performance during exercise and the point of termination of the exercise bout [2]. Accordingly, as the definition of the term has changed, so too has its use as a descriptor of the regulation of exercise intensity; which in part may contribute to the controversy surrounding the mechanisms associated with fatigue [3, 4]. Despite this debate, identifying exercise termination in laboratory environments is a relatively simple procedure, as the athlete exercises until volitional cessation. However, in field-based exercise, discounting medical incidents, a point of termination normally relates to the end of a game or event. As such, the absence of a clear exercise termination point during field-based exercise clouds the understanding of the existence and potential mechanisms responsible for fatigue. Rather, the reduction in exercise intensity throughout any given match seems to represent a pattern of regulation of intensity, rather than classic notions of fatigue *per se*. Given the mechanisms underlying fatigue are likely to be duration and intensity dependent [1, 2], the model of exercise used will somewhat dictate the conclusions reached. Accordingly, while laboratory research is presented as evidence for fatigue-causing physiological mechanisms, the lack of specificity to field-based activities often reduces the application of these findings to the field.

Given most team sport participants do not fail to finish a match, the term fatigue is often used to describe the transient or progressive reduction in work rate during an athletic event [5-7]. Compounding the use of the term fatigue in field environments, is that the self-selected nature of field-based exercise results in stochastic fluctuations in exercise intensity which makes quantifying fatigue difficult. Moreover, the self-selected nature of field-based exercise also mitigates the applicability of many laboratory findings sought by athletes, coaches and scientists in the field. That said, during most (continuous) prolonged, endurance events in the field, the measurement of speed or power output is not difficult to obtain and can provide descriptive data as to the regulation of exercise intensity [8]. However, during team sports where the exercise patterns consist of prolonged, high intensity, intermittent activities, the quantification of fatigue and exercise regulation is somewhat more problematic.

Until recently, the quantification of field-based, team sport physical demands was a laborious and protracted situation, often involving video and time-motion analysis of individual players [9-11]. More recently the use of equipment such as Global Positioning Systems (GPS) and semi-automated digital image tracking systems technology has expedited this process without sacrificing accuracy or reliability [12-14]. As such, recent advancements in technology have allowed an unprecedented ability to monitor and measure physical performance directly from team sport competitions [15-23]. Armed with the knowledge and data collected from a variety of team sports, it is possible to further explore the presence of 'fatigue', or more appropriately, the regulation of exercise workloads, during field-based intermittent-sprint exercise. A deeper evaluation of the regulation of exercise workloads during matches may also allow greater appreciation of the intensity- and duration-specific mechanisms likely to affect physical performance of team sport athletes. Accordingly, the use of quasi-experimental procedures for field-based sports may further allow for the development of a more refined model that explains the impact of fatigue on team sport exercise.

To date, most evidence for the mechanisms causing fatigue for team sport exercise have been extrapolated from laboratory simulations of intermittent-sprint exercise, and relate to a mixture of biochemical, neurological and central perturbations [24, 25]. However, many laboratory simulations have little resemblance of exercise patterns or technical skill demands evident in team sport games, and generally involve externally fixed-intensities preventing the incorporation self-selected pacing strategies [26]. Given the importance of mechanisms of fatigue being intensity- and duration-specific, the lack of ecological validity of many laboratory protocols may mislead the understanding of how exercise is regulated in the field. That said, the replication of game-based exercise patterns in laboratory surrounds is problematic due to the infinite permutations of activities incorporated in any team sport game. Accordingly, given the improved technology to track player movements, larger samples can now be measured and therefore the analysis of these data can provide evidence for the game-specific regulation of exercise intensity.

Therefore, given the debate regarding the mechanisms of fatigue in (team sport) athletes, the lack of ecological validity of laboratory protocols to replicate field-based exercise and the improvement in player tracking technology, this chapter will discuss the presence and extent of fatigue in team sport exercise and the potential underlying physiological mechanisms. Included in this discussion will be a summary of recent literature on motion analysis of team sports, field-based physiological measures associated with motion-analysis data, and the effect of extraneous environments on the physiology and motion patterns of team sport games. Collectively, these various sets of data and research findings will be used to provide hypotheses on the role and effect of various physiological mechanisms potentially responsible for the regulation of exercise intensity during game-based, team sport exercise.

Game-based Motion Patterns as Indicators of Exercise Regulation and Fatigue

Most field-based team sports are primarily aerobic sports that demand that athletes complete irregular bouts of high-intensity activity. The work demands are very stochastic, often require unorthodox movement patterns and are completed with varying and unpredictable recovery periods. In addition to these, players are also required to complete sports-specific technical skills such as kicking, passing, throwing, jumping, catching, tackling, hitting etc. Due to these unpredictable physical demands, the patterns of exercise intensity are difficult to model precisely.

The first studies of time-motion in team sports used labour intensive methods such as pen-and-paper tracking on a scaled map [27, 28] or video-based analysis [9, 29] that only allowed for single players to be tracked at one time. Because of the labour intensive nature of these methods, such studies were typically restricted to universities or research institutes. Due to these limitations, the precise understanding of physical demands in competition was relatively poor. Nonetheless, these methods provided the early information from which the current understanding of fatigue patterns in team sports is based.

The most common method used for analysing game-based movement patterns has required the players to be individually filmed from the side of the field and then later analysed during play back where coding of pre-defined activities took place [6, 30-38]. More recently, the quantification of exercise intensity and distribution of physical demands within team sports has been simplified for the end user with the development of sophisticated semi-automated computer-based match analysis systems (e.g. ProZone, Amisco, SICS) and portable microtechnology including GPS [12, 14, 39]. Many of these systems now permit scientists to monitor the movement characteristics of each player, officials and the ball during matches. Indeed, these systems have lead to a recent increase in the number of sophisticated analysis of the exercise intensity and movement patterns in various team sports [13, 15-18, 20, 21, 23, 40-42].

With the change in technology and improvements in measurement precision, a clearer understanding of movement patterns and physical demands is developing [10]. Until recently, most of the focus of the in-match performance measures for identifying fatigue had been on changes in the global measures of exercise intensity (i.e. total distance travelled) and/or higher intensity activities (i.e. high-intensity running (HIR) and sprint performance) [6, 7, 9, 31, 43-46]. From these measures, both 'cumulative' and 'transient' fatigue has been identified during match play [7]. In addition, recent studies have also identified that there may be more complex changes in the lower and moderate-intensity activities that occur to preserve the ability to achieve high-intensity exercise during critical periods of play, even during the final stages of matches [18, 19, 47].

Cumulative Fatigue

The first observations of fatigue from match analysis were reported as reductions in total distance (TD) covered during the second half of matches. For example, Carling et al. [11] recently reported that the typical reduction in distance travelled in each half of elite level soccer matches was -3.1% (range -9.4 to +0.8%). These results agree with reports from many other team sports that have shown TD to be reduced in the second half in a variety of team sports including rugby league [48], Australian Rules Football [18], soccer officials [49], rugby union [22]. If considered in isolation, it can be interpreted that cumulative fatigue occurs during team sport match play.

Unfortunately, a global description of the changes in TD travelled between halves during games does not provide specific insight into how exercise intensity is regulated by team sport players. Many authors have reported that HIR distances (i.e. >14−15 $km \cdot h^{-1}$) are critical for performance in football codes and that the ability to defend reductions in these variables are important for success [6, 7, 31]. Therefore, many investigators have examined how HIR patterns change during matches to gain a better understanding of fatigue in team sport matches.

As evidence of 'cumulative' fatigue during team sport match play, Mohr et al. [6] reported that the distance travelled with HIR was significantly reduced in the second half compared to the first during international soccer matches. These authors also reported that HIR distance was 35–45% lower in the final 15 min of the match compared to the first 15 min. More recently, Rampinini et al. [15] showed that elite level players who completed more HIR during the first half of Premier League soccer matches had the greatest reduction in HIR during the second half. In this study, the mean reduction in HIR (~100 m) from the first to the second half accounted for approximately 25% in the reduction of total distance (~400 m) during the second half of the match. Similarly, Coutts et al. [18] also reported that ~49% of the reduction in total distance travelled from the first to the second half in Australian Rules football was also from HIR. Collectively, these examples show that reductions in both TD and HIR distance measures in team sports can be used to show 'cumulative' fatigue. Notably, a relatively small proportion of the reduction in TD is attributed to higher intensity activities, indicating that changes in lower intensity activities may also be important indicators of fatigue in team sports.

Transient Fatigue

Many studies have also shown that 'transient' fatigue occurs during team sport matches [6, 17, 18]. For example, Mohr et al. [6] used manual video-based time-motion analysis to first show that the amount of HIR in the 5-min period immediately after the most intense 5-min interval during international level soccer matches were of lower intensity than the average match intensity. Similarly, Bradley et al. [17] extended this observation using more accurate semi-automated match analysis procedures on the English Premier League soccer to show that the amount of HIR decreased by ~50% in the 5-min following the most intense 5-min period of match play; and further, that time between each HIR bout increased as the match progressed. Indeed, it was reported that the recovery times between each HIR bout was increased by 28% from the first 15-min period of Premier League soccer matches to the last. Finally, Coutts et al. [18] demonstrated using a median split technique, that the players who completed most HIR during each quarter of professional level Australian Rules Football had a significantly greater reduction in HIR during the subsequent quarter than the players that completed less HIR. Collectively, these findings show that 'transient' fatigue can occur following intense exercise periods during team sport matches.

Despite evidence that both the ‘cumulative’ and the ‘transient’ fatigue occurs in matches, it still seems that players retain the capacity to achieve peak speeds when required. For example, Duffield et al. [19] demonstrated that the amount of very high-intensity running (i.e. >20 $km \cdot h^{-1}$) and the peak speeds achieved during each sprint effort did not change in the last quarter of Australian Rules Football matches. Additionally, Bradley et al. [17] reported no change in peak sprint velocities during English Premier League soccer matches in players (N=370) from any playing position when the match was analysed in 15-min periods. Moreover, many other studies have shown that the amount to sprint distance reduces towards the end of matches [6, 7, 31, 32], especially in players from positions that require more sprinting early in matches [17, 21]. Nonetheless, it is interesting that although both 'transient' and 'cumulative' fatigue are increasingly apparent in most team sports as matches progress [18, 50], many players can preserve the ability to reach peak speeds, even toward the end of matches [11, 17]. This ability to maintain peak sprint efforts despite evidence of cumulative fatigue may also be due to pacing strategies adopted during match play.

Lower and Moderate-Intensity Activities

Lower intensity activities (LIA) such as standing still, walking, jogging and running comprises the majority (up to 92%) of team sport match play [51], and these lower intensity efforts allow the athlete to recover between HIR bouts. Indeed, it has been suggested that LIA influence the quality of HIA during team sport competition and therefore are important to the outcome of the match [52-54]. Moreover, some authors have suggested that match-related fatigue may also be identified through changes in the LIA profile [18-20, 45]. It may be that players choose to carry out fewer activities at lower or moderate intensities (i.e. <15 km·h^{-1}) and also select to move at a slower rate between each high-intensity effort as matches continue and fatigue ensues. This 'pacing' may allow players to conserve energy for critical moments in the match, as these critical moments can occur unpredictably, demanding maximal efforts.

In support of this suggestion, several studies have shown that team sport athletes reduce the velocities at which they travel within the lower and moderate speed zones as matches progress [18-20, 45, 55]. For example, Duffield et al. [19] reported that both the HIR (<14.4 km·h^{-1}) and moderate-intensity activities (MIA: 7.0−14.4 km·h^{-1}) were reduced, whilst velocities at very high-intensities (>20 km·h^{-1}) were maintained in 10 professional Australian Rules Football players during preseason matches played in hot conditions. Similarly, Castagna et al. [45] reported no between-half effect for HIR, despite a significant MIR (8−13 km·h^{-1}) decrement during the second half in young (under 12 y) soccer players during match play. More recently, Coutts et al. [18] showed that while TD and HIR travelled were reduced following the first quarter of professional Australian Rules Football, the average speeds travelled during LIA (i.e. <14.4 km·h^{-1}) were reduced but the average speeds achieved in the HIR zones (i.e. >14.4 km·h^{-1}) were not affected. Moreover, Rampinini et al. [15] demonstrated that the majority (~80%) of the decrease in TD during the second half of Premier League soccer matches was through decreases in distance spent travelling below 14.4 km·h^{-1}. Combined, these examples show that it is not only the distances travelled at higher intensity activities that show reduction during team sport matches. It seems that the distances travelled during lower-intensity activities are often down regulated as a match progresses. It is possible that this occurs in order to defend the ability to achieve high-intensities when required later in the match.

In summary, the general findings from time-motion studies from team sports during match play show that fatigue manifests in different forms during matches. There are two commonly defined signs of fatigue during match play: 1) 'cumulative' fatigue which is represented by a reduction in TD travelled as a match progresses, and 2) 'transient' fatigue which is represented by a momentary or period of reduced exercise intensity (usually following a period of increased exercise intensity). There are also indicators of the adoption of pacing strategies that occur during team sport match play. Indeed, it has recently been suggested that players might alter their physical activity during team sport match play on the basis of both pre-match contexts (e.g. prior experience in similar circumstances, fitness levels, match importance) and physiological alterations during the game (internal temperature, muscle metabolite accumulation, and substrate availability) to protect the ability to perform at higher intensities toward the end of the game [47]. This theory could explain the frequently occurring patterns in time-motion profile of team sports. Certainly, there is now evidence to suggest that changes in lower and moderate intensity activities appear to also be of some importance [18, 19]. It might be that changes in distances travelled in lower and moderate-intensity speed zones may represent self-preservation for later involvement in critical events during a match. Nonetheless, caution must be taken when interpreting these results as we have used game-based examples from a large variety of sports that are completed over varying durations and diverse technical/tactical requirements. Therefore, we suggest that where possible any diagnosis of fatigue time-motion measures should be interpreted in conjunction with other psycho-biological measures.

GAME-BASED PHYSIOLOGICAL RESPONSES AS INDICATORS OF PHYSIOLOGICAL STATE

Central to arguments regarding the mechanisms causing fatigue is the resultant physiological state that may precipitate or identify potential fatigue-inducing agents [25]. In particular, this often relates to the physiological perturbations in the exercising musculature creating or promoting a fatigued state; thereby restricting muscular contraction and resulting in a reduction in work performed [37]. While sufficient laboratory evidence exists to discredit many physiological perturbations as being fatigue causing agents [2, 5], little field-based data exists to describe the physiological state of an athlete matched to the measured work performed during a game. As such, given the research focus on physiological markers of fatigue, it is pertinent to describe the physiological responses to team sport games, supplementing motion-analysis data, to describe both the work performed and the physiological state of team sport athletes.

Energy Substrate Depletion

Not surprisingly, prolonged intermittent-sprint sports, such as football or soccer, result in a significant depletion of intramuscular carbohydrate stores. Muscle biopsy data collected from high-performance national level players during simulated matches indicates a progressive reduction in muscle glycogen during the match, with post-game reductions as much as 50% [25, 37]. In particular, the predominant depletion of glycogen occurs in the type I fibers (50% empty or nearly empty), with smaller reductions (20 - 40% nearly empty) in type II fibers [37, 56]. Despite a continued reduction in muscle glycogen stores over the 90 min of a soccer match, muscle lactate values remain relatively stable (~20 ± 10 $mmol \cdot kg^{-1}$d.w), although these values show high variability due to the sampling time during the match and exercise performed prior to sampling. Similarly, muscle pH shows a substantial reduction over the duration of the first half of a soccer match, becoming as low as ~6.9; however, by the end of the match, muscle pH has returned to near pre-match values [25]. Accordingly, the intermittent-nature of team sports has been shown to be taxing on glycolytic and oxidative energy pathways, and as such substantial carbohydrate depletion exists following team sport matches.

Given the evidence for the bioenergetic requirements of prolonged intermittent-sprint exercise and substantial muscle carbohydrate depletion, it is also not surprising to observe sustained, elevated metabolite values [7, 25]. Data from several sports including Australian Rules Football, rugby union and soccer indicate blood lactate values of 6–10 $mmol \cdot L^{-1}$ [7, 19, 57]. Additionally, as with muscle pH values, blood pH data indicates a reduction in pH over the duration of a soccer match, along with reductions in blood buffering agents such as bicarbonate [58]. Moreover, measures of blood glucose and triglycerides indicate a gradual reduction and increment, respectively as the match progresses [25, 37]. The opposing nature of the glucose and triglyceride blood responses highlights the gradual reduction in muscle glycogen stores as intermittent-sprint exercise continues, while the reliance on free fatty acids increases. These data further develop the picture that prolonged intermittent-sprint sports heavily tax all energy substrate utilisation pathways.

As highlighted earlier, the distances covered and mean speeds of the different intensity zones are reduced as a match progresses [18]. Whether the change in substrate utilisation is a consequence or cause of the reduction in volume and intensity of exercise is unknown. Together these data suggest that the energetic load of intermittent-sprint exercise involved in team-sports is substantial, which may have some bearing on the ensuing development of fatigue.

Cardiovascular and Thermoregulatory Responses

The prolonged, intermittent nature of most team sports is well known to impose a significant load on the cardiovascular system, from a combination of elevated cardiovascular demands, a hypohydrated state and rise in internal body temperatures [59]. Data collected during soccer, rugby and Australian Rules Football matches indicates mean heart rate responses of between 75 – 85% max; however, as expected with the intermittent nature of these sports, heart rates can range from 65% to maximal [57, 60]. While logistics of data collection prevent the measurement of VO_2 during competitive environments, the transient nature of near maximal heart rate values is likely to indicate that inability to maintain the aerobic or cardiovascular load is not a direct cause of fatigue [61]. However, the elevated heart rate responses, often in the presence of reduced volumes of work, during latter periods of a match would suggest the development of cardiovascular drift due to loss of blood volume [62].

The hydration status of team sport athletes is a popular topic within the exercise sciences, with a large volume of research on hydration responses to intermittent-sprint exercise and training sessions [63]. A range of laboratory studies highlight the negative effects of hypohydration [62], although the extent of this relationship is currently being challenged [47]. A handful of studies from competitive environments describe the change in mass before and after a match [19, 64]. Normal post-game reductions in body mass of players is around 2 – 3 kg, resulting in a fluid loss rate of 1 – 2 $kg{\cdot}h^{-1}$, depending on match duration and environmental conditions [65]. However the quantification of fluid consumption during a match is normally difficult to measure, and not reported. Further, post-game hydration status is rarely reported, although has been shown to be >1.020 Urine Specific Gravity [19, 64]. Although there is likely to be a significant reduction in blood volume, resulting in a hypohydrated state following a match, recent research has questioned the causative role of this type of physiological change in the development of fatigue [66, 67]. Rather than hypohydration being a cause of fatigue *per se*, it has been highlighted as having a role in reducing the ability to tolerate an increasing internal thermal load during exercise [67].

Despite the plethora of literature highlighting the dangers of dehydration and risk of heat illness [68, 69], there is relatively little research describing thermoregulatory responses to match-play in sports. To date, only a handful of studies report core or muscle temperature for team sport matches, [33, 70], and even less in hot environmental conditions where the thermoregulatory system is more likely to be taxed [19]. From these early data, it seems that core temperature is rarely elevated for any length of time above 39.5°C, and when it is, it is usually accompanied by a reduction in work, resulting in a reduction or maintenance of internal temperatures within tolerable limits [67, 71]. Further, while muscle temperature is often elevated to 40°C, as expected, it rarely exceeds these upper limits and has been reported as beneficial for match performance to remain elevated [33]. However, given the limited published data on these thermoregulatory variables collected during competitive environments, definitive statements on the thermoregulatory responses to team sport exercise are difficult. Consequently, the prolonged maintenance of elevated internal temperatures during team sports, while adding to the cardiovascular and thermoregulatory load, even in hot conditions, seems to be maintained within tolerable limits.

Neuromuscular Responses

Previously we have reported the lack of reduction in peak speeds, and minimal change in mean velocities in the higher intensity zones towards the latter stages of team sport matches [18]. However, post-exercise measures of neuromuscular power indicate a small, but potentially important suppression of peak power, such as 2 cm in peak vertical jump height [72]. Further, repeated 30-m sprint times have been reported to be 2 – 3% slower following match-play [33]. These data are somewhat in opposition to GPS data indicating that peak match speeds are not slower as the match progresses, although this may be evidence that either peak velocities are not reached during competitive environments or the motivation to perform post-game is suppressed.

To date, few studies report voluntary activation during and following prolonged match-play in intermittent-sprint sports. Girard et al. [73] reported a reduction in both voluntary and centrally activated maximal force production following 3 h of tennis match-play. While the duration of tennis match-play exceeds most other team sports, even by 150 min of play, reductions in both voluntary and evoked force productions were present. Accordingly, this may indicate that following prolonged, intermittent-sprint sports, force production is suppressed via both voluntary and central mechanisms, highlighting some role for both peripheral and centrally-mediated processes of fatigue [74].

Summary of Physiological State of Team Sport Athlete

In summary, while many time-motion studies show minimal reduction in peak velocities throughout competitive matches, a significant reduction in distance covered at both moderate-to-low and high velocities is present. Concurrently, there are small but prominent reductions in voluntary and evoked neuromuscular force production. Further, the post-match physiological state of a team sport athlete includes, a prominent depletion of intra-muscular glycogen stores, elevated intramuscular and blood metabolites, elevated muscle and core temperatures and reduced blood volumes from evaporative sweat loss resulting in a state of hypohydration. Despite the pronounced physiological perturbations resulting from prolonged team sport matches, it would not seem evident that the change in any of these singular factors would be a direct causative factor associated with fatigue. Consequently, it may be the combination of a multitude of these physiological changes that results in the regulation of exercise intensity observed during team sport matches.

Effects of Altered Conditions on the Regulation of Exercise; Effects of the Heat

The discussion of motion analysis patterns and the physiological state of team sport athletes assists the development of a clearer picture of the regulation of game-based exercise intensity. However, by supplementing this situation with the addition of a superimposed external condition known to result in the earlier development of fatigue, such as exercise in the heat [75], also helps develop an understanding of the potential underlying mechanisms of fatigue.

Exercise in warm to hot conditions is well known to exacerbate the physiological stress of the bout, while also resulting in an earlier onset of fatigue and exercise termination [59, 75]. In particular, high environmental temperatures are generally related to a less efficient thermoregulatory system; whereby exercise results in higher sweat losses, reduced blood volume, increased cardiovascular load and higher core temperatures than in cooler conditions [62]. The increased physiological load has traditionally been associated with the earlier onset of fatigue, however may not necessarily be a direct cause of the reduction in exercise performance [76, 77]. Recent evidence highlights that although the physiological systems encounter a greater load in the heat, the observed reduction in exercise intensity is evident before systems become critically overloaded [77, 78]. Accordingly, either as a response to a more rapid rise in the physiological load [75], in anticipation of the growing physiological load [76] or a greater perception of load and effort [3], muscle recruitment is altered thus reducing exercise performance. Moreover, it is thought that this reduction in recruitment of exercising musculature is a protective mechanism to control heat generation, and limit the rise in core temperature [76, 79]. However, while an abundance of laboratory-based research findings exist on this topic, there is a dearth of literature reporting what occurs in field-based environments, particularly for team sports.

A small number of studies report core temperature responses to team sport games in cool (<18°C) conditions [33, 47], but do not report any measures of match physical demands. A recent study reported player motion activities alongside thermoregulatory data for elite pre-season Australian Rules Football games in hot (30°C) conditions [19]. The findings of this study highlighted some interesting trends that add to the picture of game-based fatigue developed in the previous sections. First, as noted earlier, as the match progressed, only small reductions in the distance covered in high-intensity zones was observed, and that the velocities of these efforts (including sprint efforts) were not reduced. Second, as the game progressed, the major reduction in distance travelled or speed of efforts occurred in the moderate-intensity zone (7–14 $km \cdot h^{-1}$). Third, that the reduction in moderate-intensity work was inversely correlated ($r= -0.88$) with a higher mid-game core temperature. Finally, core temperature responses reached a plateau after the first 30 min, with only minimal increases as the game continued (final core temperatures were 39.3 ± 0.4°C). Accordingly, it seems possible that the effects of hot environmental conditions predominantly result in the down regulation of moderate to low-intensity efforts that may not be directly critical to game performance.

While the limited evidence does suggest altered game-based pacing strategies and motion activities due to the heat, the amelioration of this superimposed condition via body cooling also assists in understanding how exercise is regulated in the field. Pre-cooling is a process whereby skin, muscle and/or core temperature is lowered prior to exercise in the heat to reduce the physiological load and improve exercise performance [80]. A range of laboratory-based studies provide evidence of the ergogenic qualities of cooling prior to exercise in the heat for prolonged continuous and intermittent-sprint exercise [79, 81]. However, to date no studies have attempted to determine the effects of pre-cooling for team sport athletes in hot conditions in the field. Recently, a field-based study incorporating pre-cooling before a free-paced exercise protocol as part of a conditioning training session showed promising results [71]. These data highlighted that a pre-cooling intervention that blunted the rise in core temperature resulted in an increased distance covered during the session, predominantly in the speed zones incorporating 10 – 16 $km \cdot h^{-1}$. While sprint speeds and distances were not different between cooled and non-cooled bouts, players selected higher workloads for the self-selected work performed between sprint efforts. Moreover, recent unpublished evidence highlights that during hot conditions, Australian Rules Football players cover a reduced distance when compared to cooler conditions [82]. The decreased distances covered during hot games, are alongside elevated core temperatures, increased sweat loss and higher perceptual exertion. Accordingly, it seems evident that team sport exercise in the heat results in a down-regulation of work performed for a similar physiological load. Additionally, the reduced workload may be predominantly evident in the moderate to hard zones of running, rather than peak speeds or very high intensity efforts.

POSSIBLE MECHANISMS RELATING TO GAME-BASED FATIGUE

Before speculating on the possible mechanisms regulating field-based exercise intensity, it is of benefit to summarise the state of knowledge thus far. Data from player time-motion analyses indicates that fatigue in team sports, in the sense of reduced physical work, manifests as a reduction in distance and velocities of lower and moderate speed zones (7 – 14 $km \cdot h^{-1}$) and to a lesser extent reductions in the higher intensity zones (14 – 30 $km \cdot h^{-1}$). These reductions in exercise intensities are alongside depletion in muscle carbohydrate stores, elevation of metabolites, prolonged cardiovascular load, increased thermoregulatory load and a small suppression of neuromuscular power. Additionally, when we superimpose warm conditions, the decrease in low-moderate intensity activity seems greater, while the change in higher intensity zones is similar to cool conditions. Further, this situation is countered in cooler environments or when pre-cooling interventions are applied to intermittent-sprint exercise in the heat. Despite these imposed loads, peak speeds may be as fast in the latter stages of a match as they are at the start. Moreover, there is little reduction in very high intensity zone distance or velocity. Within the contextual demands of intermittent, high-intensity efforts over a prolonged duration, fatigue in team sports may not be thought of as a classical decline in performance until an inability to continue. Rather, physical fatigue in team sports may be better represented by the gradual down-regulation of exercise in the moderate and lower intensity zones; either to protect or continue work in the higher zones which may have more relevance to match performance.

The regulation of exercise intensity to ensure ability to perform near maximal work at the end of a match represents the use of pacing strategies to ensure successful completion. Pacing strategies have gained some attention in the research literature for prolonged, continuous modes of exercise, such as cycling and running [83]. It is often noted in long distance events that athletes may finish with a fast spurt of higher intensity activity [83, 84]. Accordingly, athletes predominantly ensure completion of an event without allowing physiological disturbances outside of (individual) tolerable homeostatic ranges [85]. These observations, when evaluated in light of the information presented here, seem apt for a description of pacing in team sports. The context of most team sports is that key match-specific performance indicators often revolve around high-intensity efforts, and the inability to perform those efforts results in overall sub-optimal performance. Thus it is possible that the understanding of the need to respond and perform near maximal efforts at intermittent time points is an overriding factor in the regulation of work between these efforts. Consequently, ensuring and protecting the ability to perform these efforts may result in conscious decision making to reduce work intensity between efforts, while ensuring physiological responses remain within tolerable limits is of non-conscious control. This interaction of physiological feedback and anticipation of future demands may explain the larger reduction in moderate zone intensities, and ability to continue to perform maximal efforts as a match progresses.

In the ecologically valid environment of field-based data collection, the context of the match is central to the decision making process regarding regulation of exercise intensity. High-intensity efforts are generally regarded as critical to match performance, and hence the ability to perform these actions late in a match can be crucial. Accordingly, this context may explain why the reduction in high-intensity zones, in both absolute and relative terms, is smaller than that observed in other intensity zones [18, 19]. When repeated high-intensity efforts are performed with minimal recovery, the resulting metabolic perturbations are likely to inhibit muscular contraction and reduce high-intensity performance [86]. Outside of these repeated high-intensity efforts, most of the reported physiological responses to team sport activity are pronounced, without being extreme. Therefore, these data may suggest that some reduction in high-intensity activities results from interruption of peripheral contractile functioning. However, to allow recovery or prevent further reductions, work rates in lower-intensity zones are reduced to facilitate faster recovery or prevent further extreme physiological changes. As an example, the interaction of factors such as reducing glycogen stores, increasing core temperature and reduced available blood volume may result in physiological and cognitive changes precipitating the adjustment of self-selected work. Moreover, the greater reductions in lower-moderate intensity zones when external environments such as hot conditions amplify the physiological load also fit with this proposed response. As such, the reduction in high-intensity zones may relate to the reduced contractile ability of the muscle, as evidenced by reductions in post-match peak power and voluntary activation [72, 73] while the reduction in moderate-intensity zones buffers further reduction in high-intensity activities and ensures physiological perturbations remain within tolerable limits. Accordingly, this somewhat ensures the ability to perform key game demands for the duration of the match and further ensure that physiological perturbations do not become catastrophic.

While this speculation of mechanisms regulating match exercise intensities has focussed on physiological responses, the role of perceptual responses in the adopted pacing strategies are also important. Although there are limited rating of perceived exertion (RPE) data reported alongside measures of work during team sport matches, free-paced exercise in laboratory conditions has been reported to be regulated based on maintaining non-maximal perceived exertion [3, 61]. Consequently, the perception of the demands at any time during a match may also influence conscious regulation of non-maximal exercise intensities at non-critical times during a match. Further, the increased perception of thermal stress and RPE normally noted in hot environments may also add to the increased perceptual load and thus the reduced work and slower pacing strategy adopted in the heat, as noted previously [82, 84]. Hence, although the control of any number of physiological responses are important factors in the regulation of self-selected exercise intensity; the perception of the current physical load, combined with an appreciation of future game demands, are also likely to be important in the regulation of match-based physical activity patterns.

In summary, ‘transient’ fatigue resulting from repeated high-intensity bouts is likely to be from an inhibition of sufficient contractile recovery. As further reductions in high-intensity work may have performance implications, it is possible these reductions correspond to peripheral rather than central factors. Accordingly, a smaller reduction in high-intensity volumes are observed as a match continues, possibly due to the conscious awareness and context of game demands. In contrast, moderate workloads are reduced to a greater extent and are more likely to result from central mechanisms. Exercise in these zones is often perceived as not as critical to match performance, and may revolve around recovery and protection of anticipated high-intensity efforts. Consequently, it is possible reductions in these zones may result from centrally-mediated mechanisms. Additionally, the perceptual load of the game, the environment, previous activity and prediction of future activity also supplements the physiological feedback regulating self-selected activity. Given the importance ascribed to high-intensity efforts, any self-selected reduction in effort is likely to be more pronounced in the moderate rather than high-intensity zones. Overall, the regulation of team sport match intensity results from a mixture of feedback on physiological state, feed-forward anticipation of future match demands, layered with perception of current and future demands. These systems are likely to be integrated to adopt the appropriate pacing strategy and regulate exercise intensity to fulfil game demands, while tolerating the imposed physiological load.

LIMITATIONS OF INTERPRETING GAME-BASED DATA

The two important areas of focus for this chapter are also the two major limiting factors in the interpretation of the reported findings; those being the use of field-based data and the use of GPS technology, respectively. First, as outlined earlier, the strength of much of the data reported here is the ecologically valid environment within which data was collected. These data represents ecologically valid physiology and performance data, and as such is not constrained by the model or mode used in simulated laboratory environments. Moreover, the predominance of laboratory data and lack of field-based data, further adds to the strength of this generally descriptive data. However, the strength of this data may also be perceived as a weakness when trying to provide mechanistic causes to any observed fatigue, or more aptly, regulation of exercise intensity. A consequence of the ecologically valid setting for much of the reported data are environments that may have a range of uncontrolled external factors: such as ground size, opposition, tactics and environment, that can also influence the results. Further, the co-ordinated, time-aligned collection of physiological data throughout matches is often difficult due to the logistics of collecting data during competition matches. As such, the lack of published data, logistical difficulties of controlling the environment for data collection and limiting the intrusion into athlete routines may limit causative findings resulting from the current collection of data.

Another limitation of the reported data is the reliance on relatively recent advances in technology to record athlete movement patterns. While GPS technology is the favoured method of data collection to quantify movement patterns in many team sports, and allows unprecedented access to measures of player movements, it is not without questions as to accuracy and reliability [14]. Recent research has reported both favourable [12] and less favourable [39] findings for the accuracy and reliability of GPS technology in sports settings. In general, the accuracy of GPS technology is highest when the exercise involves longer duration, slower movements and limited change in direction (<5%). Unfortunately, team sports can rarely be described by the above conditions, and hence higher velocity movements and repeated changes in direction result in a reduction in GPS accuracy [14, 39]. Accordingly, the largest variance in GPS measures is observed at the very high-intensity zones (20 - 30%). However, when the same device is worn on the same player, the intra-device reliability is acceptable to compare between conditions or sessions [14].

As such, GPS technology is likely to under-record distance covered, particularly within the higher intensity zones; although there is no evidence to indicate these errors change with the duration of data collection [12, 14]. A further consideration is also the lack of use of accelerometer measures to quantify high-intensity efforts over short durations that do not reach speeds classified as "high-intensity". As yet, fast accelerations that do not last more than 1 - 2 s are not factored into high-intensity measures, although this is likely to change as technology improves the resolution of measures [39]. Consequently, the use of GPS technology to quantify match movement patterns is still in its infancy and will improve with improved technology.

A final limitation to be considered is the predominant research focus on the football codes as the medium to collect and report field-based data. Given a central tenant of field-based research is to avoid the constraints imposed by the exercise model used in a laboratory, to then expect conclusions made from team sport data to suit all sports is somewhat hypocritical. Accordingly, as the duration or intensity of the sport in focus change, so too will the likely mechanisms that result in the reduction of performance or fatigue.

CONCLUSION

In this chapter we have examined the patterns of exercise regulation during team sport competition and attempted to identify fatigue from these patterns. Accordingly, we have described that both 'cumulative' and 'transient' fatigue occurs during these sports in competitive environments. Further, we have also postulated on the possible underlying mechanisms responsible for fatigue and discussed the possibility of subconscious pacing of players during team sport exercise. Based on the collection of available field-based data, it is suggested that there may be a complex regulatory system including a number of psycho-biological processes that may act to influence the pacing of physical efforts during matches. This pacing effect may allow players to conserve effort in anticipation of ensuing high-intensity responses to game demands. Clearly this contention needs to be tested experimentally, and therefore we suggest that further field-based studies are conducted to provide greater ecological validity to studies examining fatigue in team based sports.

REFERENCES

[1] Enoka RM, Stuart DG. Neurobiology of muscle fatigue. *J Appl Physiol*, 1992, 72, 1631-48.

[2] Enoka RM, Duchateau J. Muscle fatigue: what, why and how it influences muscle function. *J Physiol*, 2008, 586, 11-23.

[3] St Clair Gibson A, Baden DA, Lambert MI, Lambert EV, Harley YX, Hampson D, et al. The conscious perception of the sensation of fatigue. *Sports Med*, 2003, 33, 167-76.

[4] Lambert EV, St Clair Gibson A, Noakes TD. Complex systems model of fatigue: integrative homoeostatic control of peripheral physiological systems during exercise in humans. *Br J Sports Med*, 2005, 39, 52-62.

[5] Noakes TD, St Clair Gibson A, Lambert EV. From catastrophe to complexity: a novel model of integrative central neural regulation of effort and fatigue during exercise in humans. *Br J Sports Med*, 2004, 38, 511-4.

[6] Mohr M, Krustrup P, Bangsbo J. Match performance of high-standard soccer players with special reference to development of fatigue. *J Sports Sci*, 2003, 21, 519-28.

[7] Mohr M, Krustrup P, Bangsbo J. Fatigue in soccer: A brief review *J Sports Sci*, 2005, 23, 593-9.

[8] Ebert TR, Martin DT, Stephens B, Withers RT. Power output during a professional men's road-cycling tour. *Int J Sports Physiol Perform*, 2006, 1, 324-35.

[9] Reilly T, Thomas V. A motion analysis of workrate in different positional roles in professional football match-play. *J Hum Movement Stud*, 1976, 2, 87-97.

[10] Dobson B, Keogh JWL. Methodological issues for the application of time-motion analysis research. *Strength Cond J*, 2007, 29, 48-55.

[11] Carling C, Bloomfield J, Nelsen L, Reilly T. The role of motion analysis in elite soccer: contemporary performance measurement techniques and work rate data. *Sports Med*, 2008, 38, 839-62.

[12] MacLeod H, Morris J, Nevill A, Sunderland C. The validity of a non-differential global positioning system for assessing player movement patterns in field hockey. *J Sports Sci*, 2009, 27, 121-8.

[13] Di Salvo V, Collins A, McNeill B, Cardinale M. Validation of Prozone ®: A new video-based performance analysis system. *Int J Perf Anal Sport*, 2006, 6, 108-19.

[14] Coutts AJ, Duffield R. Validity and reliability of GPS units for measuring movement demands of team sports. *J Sci Med Sport*, 2010, 13, 133-135.

[15] Rampinini E, Coutts AJ, Castagna C, Sassi R, Impellizzeri FM. Variation in top level soccer match performance. *Int J Sports Med*, 2007, 28, 1018-24.

[16] Rampinini E, Impellizzeri FM, Castagna C, Coutts AJ, Wisløff U. Technical performance during soccer matches of the Italian Serie A league: effect of fatigue and competitive level. *J Sci Med Sport*, 2009, 12, 227-33.

[17] Bradley PS, Sheldon W, Wooster B, Olsen P, Boanas P, Krustrup P. High-intensity running in FA Premier League soccer matches. *J Sports Sci*, 2009, 27, 159-68.

[18] Coutts AJ, Quinn J, Hocking J, Castagna C, Rampinini E. Match running demands of elite Australian Rules Football. *J Sci Med Sport*, 2009, doi:10.1016/j.jsams.2009.09.004.

[19] Duffield R, Coutts AJ, Quinn J. Core temperature responses and match running performance during intermittent-sprint exercise competition in warm conditions. *J Strength Cond Res*, 2009, 23, 1238-44.

[20] Di Salvo V, Baron R, Tschan H, Calderon Montero FJ, Bachl N, Pigozzi F. Performance characteristics according to playing position in elite soccer. *Int J Sports Med*, 2007, 28, 222-7.

[21] Di Salvo V, Gregson W, Atkinson G, Tordoff P, Drust B. Analysis of high intensity activity in Premier League soccer. *Int J Sports Med*, 2009, 30, 205-12.

[22] Roberts SP, Trewartha G, Higgitt RJ, El-Abd J, Stokes KA. The physical demands of elite English rugby union. *J Sports Sci*, 2008, 26, 825-33.

[23] Sykes D, Twist C, Hall S, Nicholas C, Lamb K. Semi-automated time-motion analysis of senior elite rugby league. *Int J Perf Anal Sport*, 2009, 9, 47-59.

[24] Reilly T, Gilbourne D. Science and football: a review of applied research in the football codes. *J Sports Sci*, 2003, 21, 693-705.

[25] Bangsbo J, Iaia FM, Krustrup P. Metabolic response and fatigue in soccer. *Int J Sports Physiol Perform*, 2007, 2, 111-27.

[26] Duffield R, Dawson B, Bishop D, Fitzsimons M, Lawrence S. Effect of wearing an ice cooling jacket on repeat sprint performance in warm/humid conditions. *Br J Sports Med*, 2003, 37, 164-9.

[27] Hahn A, Taylor N, Hunt B, Woodhouse T, Schultz G. Physiological relationships between training activities and match play in Australian Football rovers. *Sports Coach*, 1979, 3, 3-8.

[28] Nettleton B, Sandstrom E. Skill and conditioning in Australian Rules football. *Aust J Phys Ed*, 1963, 29, 17-30.

[29] Saltin B. Metabolic fundamentals in exercise. *Med Sci Sports Exerc*, 1973, 5, 137-46.

[30] Bangsbo J, Nørregaard L, Thosøe F. Activity profile of competition soccer. *Can J Sport Sci*, 1991, 16, 110-6.

[31] Mohr M, Ellingsgaard H, Andersson H, Bangsbo J, Krustrup P. Physical demands in high-level female soccer - application of fitness tests to evaluate match performance. *J Sports Sci*, 2003, 22, 552-3.

[32] Mohr M, Krustrup P, Andersson H, Kirkendal D, Bangsbo J. Match activities of elite women soccer players at different performance levels. *J Strength Cond Res*, 2008, 22, 341-9.

[33] Mohr M, Krustrup P, Nybo L, Nielsen JJ, Bangsbo J. Muscle temperature and sprint performance during soccer matches - beneficial effect of re-warm-up at half time. *Scand J Med Sci Sports*, 2004, 14, 152-62.

[34] Krustrup P, Bangsbo J. Physiological demands of top-class soccer refereeing in relation to physical capacity: effect of intense intermittent exercise training. *J Sports Sci*, 2001, 19, 881-91.

[35] Krustrup P, Mohr M, Bangsbo J. Activity profile and physiological demands of top-class soccer assistant refereeing in relation to training status. *J Sports Sci*, 2002, 20, 861-71.

[36] Krustrup P, Mohr M, Ellingsgaard H, Bangsbo J. Physical demands during an elite female soccer game: importance of training status. *Med Sci Sports Exerc*, 2005, 37, 1242-8.

[37] Krustrup P, Mohr M, Steensberg A, Bencke J, Kjaer M, Bangsbo J. Muscle and blood metabolites during a soccer game: implications for sprint performance. *Med Sci Sports Exerc*, 2006, 38, 1165-74.

[38] Impellizzeri FM, Marcora SM, Castagna C, Reilly T, Sassi A, Iaia FM, et al. Physiological and performance effects of generic versus specific aerobic training in soccer players. *Int J Sports Med*, 2006, 27, 483-92.

[39] Duffield R, Reid M, Baker J, Spratford W. Accuracy and reliability of GPS devices for measurement of movement patterns in confined spaces for court-based sports. *J Sci Med Sport*, 2009.

[40] Rampinini E, Bishop D, Marcora SM, Ferrari Bravo D, Sassi R, Impellizzeri FM. Validity of simple field tests as indicators of match-related physical performance in top-level professional soccer players. *Int J Sports Med*, 2007, 28, 228-37.

[41] Weston M, Castagna C, Impellizzeri FM, Rampinini E, Abt G. Analysis of physical match performance in English Premier League soccer referees with particular reference to first half and player work rates. *J Sci Med Sport*, 2007, 10, 390-7.

[42] Weston M, Castagna C, Impellizzeri FM, Rampinini E, Breivik S. Ageing and physical match performance in English Premier League soccer referees. *J Sci Med Sport*, 2008, doi:10.1016/j.jsams.2008.07.009

[43] Castagna C, Abt GA, D'Ottavio S. Relation between fitness tests and match performance in elite Italian soccer referees. *J Strength Cond Res*, 2002, 16, 231-5.

[44] Castagna C, Abt GA, D'Ottavio S. The relationship between selected blood lactate thresholds and match performance in elite soccer referees. *J Strength Cond Res*, 2002, 16, 623-7.

[45] Castagna C, D'Ottavio S, Abt G. Activity profile of young soccer players during actual match play. *J Strength Cond Res*, 2003, 17, 775-80.

[46] Coutts AJ, Reaburn PRJ. Time and motion analysis of the AFL field umpire. *J Sci Med Sport*, 2000, 3, 132-9.

[47] Edwards AM, Noakes TD. Dehydration: cause of fatigue or sign of pacing in elite soccer? *Sports Med*, 2009, 39, 1-13.

[48] Sirotic AC, Coutts AJ, Knowles H, Catterick C. A comparison of match demands between elite and semi-elite rugby league competition. *J Sports Sci*, 2009, 27, 203-11.

[49] Castagna C, Abt G, D'Ottavio S. Physiological aspects of soccer refereeing performance and training. *Sports Med*, 2007, 37, 625-46.

[50] Bangsbo J. Variations in running speeds and recovery time after a sprint during top-class soccer matches. *Med Sci Sports Exerc*, 2005, 37, s87.

[51] Bangsbo J, Norregaard L, Thorso F. Activity profile of competition soccer. *Can J Sport Sci*, 1991, 16, 110-6.

[52] Bangsbo J. The physiology of soccer--with special reference to intense intermittent exercise. *Acta Physiol Scand Suppl*, 1994, 619, 1-155.

[53] Bogdanis GC, Nevill ME, Boobis LH, Lakomy HK. Contribution of phosphocreatine and aerobic metabolism to energy supply during repeated sprint exercise. *J Appl Physiol*, 1996, 80, 876-84.

[54] Gaitanos GC, Williams C, Boobis LH, Brooks S. Human muscle metabolism during intermittent maximal exercise. *J Appl Physiol*, 1993, 75, 712-9.

[55] Castagna C, Impellizzeri F, Cecchini E, Rampinini E, Alvarez JC. Effects of intermittent-endurance fitness on match performance in young male soccer players. *J Strength Cond Res*, 2009, 23, 1954-9.

[56] Bangsbo J, Mohr M, Krustrup P. Physical and metabolic demands of training and match-play in the elite football player. *J Sports Sci*, 2006, 24, 665-74.

[57] Coutts AJ, Reaburn PRJ, Abt GA. Heart rate, blood lactate concentrations, and estimated energy expenditure in a semi-professional rugby league team during match play: A case study. *J Sports Sci*, 2003, 21, 97-103.

[58] Minett G, Duffield R, Bird SP. Effects of acute multi-nutrient supplementation on rugby union game performance and recovery. *Int J Sports Physiol Perform*, 2010, in press.

[59] Reilly T, Drust B, Gregson W. Thermoregulation in elite athletes. *Curr Opin Clin Nutr Metab Care*, 2006, 9, 666-71.

[60] Ali A, Farrally M. Recording soccer players' heart rates during matches. *J Sports Sci*, 1991, 9, 183-9.

[61] Hampson DB, St Clair Gibson A, Lambert MI, Noakes TD. The influence of sensory cues on the perception of exertion during exercise and central regulation of exercise performance. *Sports Med*, 2001, 31, 935-52.

[62] Sawka MN, Latzka WA, Montain SJ, Cadarette BS, Kolka MA, Kraning II KK, et al. Physiologic tolerance to uncopensable heat: intermittent exercise, field vs laboratory. *Med Sci Sports Exerc*, 2001, 33, 422-30.

[63] Kilding AE, Tunstall H, Wraith E, Good M, Gammon C, Smith C. Sweat rate and sweat electrolyte composition in international female soccer players during game specific training. *Int J Sports Med*, 2009, 30, 443-7.

[64] Al-Jaser TA, Hasan AA. Fluid loss and body composition of elite Kuwaiti soccer players during a soccer match. *J Sports Med Phys Fit*, 2006, 46, 281-5.

[65] Shirreffs SM, Aragon-Vargas LF, Chamorro M, Maughan RJ, Serratosa L, Zachwieja JJ. The sweating response of elite professional soccer players to training in the heat. *Int J Sports Med*, 2005, 26, 90-5.

[66] Watt MJ, Garnham AP, Febbraio MA, Hargreaves M. Effect of acute plasma volume expansion on thermoregulation and exercise performance in the heat. *Med Sci Sports Exerc*, 2000, 32, 958-62.

[67] Marino FE, Cannon J, Kay D. Neuromuscular responses to hydration in moderate to warm ambient conditions during self-paced high intensity exercise. *Br J Sports Med*, 2010, 44, 961-967.

[68] Sawka MN. Physiological consequences of hypohydration: Exercise performance and thermoregulation. *Med Sci Sports Exerc*, 1992, 24, 657-70.

[69] Galloway SDR. Dehydration, rehydration, and exercise in the heat: Rehydration strategies for athletic competition. *Can J Appl Physiol*, 1999, 24, 188-200.

[70] Edwards AM, Clark NA. Thermoregulatory observations in soccer match play: professional and recreational level applications using an intestinal pill system to measure core temperature. *Br J Sports Med*, 2006, 40, 133-8.

[71] Duffield R, Steinbacher G, Fairchild TJ. The use of mixed-method, part-body pre-cooling procedures for team-sport athletes training in the heat. *J Strength Cond Res*, 2010, 23, 2524-2532.

[72] Cormack SJ, Newton RU, McGuigan MR. Neuromuscular and endocrine responses of elite players to an Australian rules football match. *Int J Sports Physiol Perform*, 2008, 3, 359–74.

[73] Girard O, Lattier G, Maffiuletti NA, Micallef JP, Millet GP. Neuromuscular fatigue during a prolonged intermittent exercise: Application to tennis. *J Electromyogr Kinesiol*, 2008, 18, 1038-46.

[74] Millet GY, Lepers R. Alterations of neuromuscular function after prolonged running, cycling and skiing exercises. *Sports Med*, 2004, 34, 105-16.

[75] Gonzalez-Alonso J, Teller C, Andersen SL, Jensen FB, Hyldig T, Nielsen B. Influence of body temperature on the development of fatigue during prolonged exercise in the heat. *J Appl Physiol*, 1999, 86, 1032-9.

[76] Marino FE. Anticipatory regulation and avoidance of catastrophe during exercise-induced hyperthermia. *Comp Biochem Physiol B Biochem Mol Biol*, 2004, 139, 561-9.

[77] Tucker R, Bester A, Lambert EV, Noakes TD, Vaughan CL, St Clair Gibson A. Non-random fluctuations in power output during self-paced exercise. *Br J Sports Med*, 2006, 40, 912-7.

[78] Nybo L. Hyperthermia and fatigue. *J Appl Physiol*, 2008, 104, 871-8.

[79] Duffield R. Cooling interventions for the protection and recovery of exercise performance from exercise-induced heat stress. *Med Sport Sci*, 2008, 53, 89-103.

[80] Marino FE. Methods, advantages, and limitations of body cooling for exercise performance. *Br J Sports Med*, 2002, 36, 89-94.

[81] Quod MJ, Martin DT, Laursen PB. Cooling athletes before competition in the heat: comparison of techniques and practical considerations. *Sports Med*, 2006, 36, 671-82.

[82] Aughey RJ, McKenna MJ. The effects of heat on AFL players during matches and training. Melbourne: Victoria University 2009.

[83] Abbiss CR, Laursen PB. Describing and understanding pacing strategies during athletic competition. *Sports Med*, 2008, 38, 239-52.

[84] St Clair Gibson A, Lambert EV, Rauch LH, Tucker R, Baden DA, Foster C, et al. The role of information processing between the brain and peripheral physiological systems in pacing and perception of effort. *Sports Med*, 2006, 36, 705-22.

[85] St Clair Gibson A, Noakes TD. Evidence for complex system integration and dynamic neural regulation of skeletal muscle recruitment during exercise in humans. *Br J Sports Med*, 2004, 38, 797-806.

[86] Spencer M, Bishop D, Dawson B, Goodman C. Physiological and metabolic responses of repeated-sprint activities:specific to field-based team sports. *Sports Med*, 2005, 35, 1025-44.

In: Regulation of Fatigue in Exercise
Editor: Frank E. Marino ISBN 978-1-61209-334-5

Chapter 8

CYTOKINE DYSREGULATION AND CANCER-RELATED FATIGUE IN EXERCISE

Jack Cannon
School of Human Movement Studies, Charles Sturt University, Bathurst NSW, Australia

ABSTRACT

Fatigue is the most frequent and severe symptom accompanying cancer and its treatment and has a significant effect on patient's functional status and quality of life. Despite this, the pathophysiological mechanisms involved in cancer-related fatigue (CRF) are yet to be fully determined. The cytokine dysregulation hypothesis has been implicated by many experts in the pathogenesis of CRF and may account for many of the symptoms accompanying cancer and its treatment. However, the relationship between cytokine dysregulation and CRF is not well established. One approach to enhance our understanding of the pathophysiological mechanisms involved in CRF may be to examine exercise-induced fatigue in cancer patients using electrophysiological and neurobiological techniques. Studies using this approach to investigate CRF are scarce, but available results demonstrate a greater contribution from central processes to the development of physical fatigue in cancer patients compared with healthy controls. Interestingly, evidence exists to suggest that cytokine dysregulation associated with cancer and its treatment may induce central fatigue through a number of different mechanisms; specifically, altered serotonin metabolism, hypothalamic-pituitary-adrenal axis dysfunction, and vagal afferent nerve activation. However, further research examining the contribution of these mechanisms are needed before any conclusions can be drawn. The results from such studies may provide new insights into the pathophysiological mechanisms involved in CRF and assist in the development of successful interventions to reduce the physiological fatigue burden in cancer patients and their carers.

INTRODUCTION

Cancer-related fatigue (CRF) is defined as a persistent sense of tiredness related to cancer and its treatment that interfers with usual functioning [1]. Fatigue is one the most prevalent symptoms experienced by cancer patients affecting 70-80% of patients during chemotherapy or radiation therapy and 30-40% of patients post-treatment across a wide variety of cancer types [2-4]. Additionally, fatigue is reported by patients to be the most frequent and severe symptom experienced and more distressing than any other symptom, including pain, nausea, and depression [5-8]. Furthermore, fatigue may be experienced for months, even years, after the completion of cancer treatment [2]. As a result, cancer patients identify fatigue as having the greatest impact on their normal activities of daily living and quality of life compared with all other symptoms [9-12]. Furthermore, CRF may also impair the timing or completion of treatment regimens, either because the extent of fatigue may limit the capacity for additional treatment or because it reduces the patient's willingness to adhere to treatment modalities [13].

Clinicians and health care providers are increasingly recognising that fatigue represents a significant consequence of cancer and its treatment. Previous studies examining CRF have primarily focused on identifying the clinical correlates accompanying fatigue burden, such as cancer type [14, 15], treatment modality [6], post-treatment duration [16], anaemia [17], depression [18, 19] and sleep disturbance [20]. However, studies examining the pathophysiological mechanisms involved in CRF are limited. This is probably because the development of CRF likely represents a complex interaction between various disease and treatment factors and patient susceptibility [21]. This is demonstrated through the lack of reliable biomarkers indicating the presence of CRF and that not all cancer patients at risk of fatigue develop significant symptoms [6, 14, 22]. The lack of research examining the mechanisms involved in CRF significantly limits our ability to develop objective diagnostic criteria and successful mechanistic-driven interventions for this deleterious symptom [21]. As such, research examining the pathophysiological mechanisms involved in CRF is a priority.

Proposed mechanisms to explain the fatigue associated with cancer and its treatment should account for associations between fatigue intensity, markers of disease burden, treatment toxicity, symptom burden, and patient behaviours [23]. In this regard, cytokine dysregulation resulting from a chronic low-grade inflammatory response has been suggested as a critical factor contributing to the pathophysiology of CRF and the development of many other deleterious symptoms typically associated with cancer and its treatment [21, 24-29]. However, studies examining the relationship between cytokine dysregulation and the presence of CRF are limited and findings are conflicting. Furthermore, the mechanistic pathways by which cytokine dysregulation may contribute to the development of CRF are poorly described. One approach to enhance our understanding of the contribution of cytokine dysregulation to the development of CRF is to examine the CRF from a known perspective; specifically, from the perspective of exercise-induced fatigue. The benefit of this approach is that the association between cytokine dyregulation and the physiological burden accompanying CRF along with the potential mechanisms involved could be objectively studied using reliable assessment methodologies widely adopted in physiological research [30].

This chapter is will provide evidence of cytokine dysregulation in cancer and its treatment and describe its association with CRF. A rationale for investigating the pathophysiological mechanisms involved in CRF through exercise-induced fatigue studies involving CRF patients will be outlined. Finally, potential pathophysiological mechanisms by which cytokine dysregulation may induce central fatigue in cancer patients will be discussed. Investigating the contribution of cytokine dysregulation to the development of CRF using exercise-induced fatigue studies may provide new insights into the pathophysiological mechanisms involved in CRF and assist in the development of successful interventions to reduce the physiological fatigue burden in cancer patients and their carers.

Evidence for Cytokine Dysregulation in the Pathophysiology of Cancer-related Fatigue

Anecdotal evidence for an association between cytokine dysregulation and chronic inflammation and CRF was first proposed based on the remarkable similarity between the general symptoms reported by cancer patients (e.g. loss of appetite, lethargy, weakness, malaise, disturbed sleep, exaggerated response to pain, and cognitive dysfunction) and the cluster of symptoms associated with cytokine-induced "sickness behaviours" [26, 31]. Sickness behaviours refers to the behavioural and physiological responses observed following the experimental or therapeutic administration of specific proinflammatory cytokines, such as Interleukin (IL)-1, IL-1β, IL-6, Interferons and Tumor Necrosis Factor (TNF)-α [32-35], and the application of agents known to induce proinflammatory responses, such as lipopolysaccharide [36, 37].

Cytokine Dysregulation in Cancer and its Treatment

The relationship between inflammation, cytokine dysregulation, cancer and its treatment is well established [38, 39]. Numerous studies examining patients with various cancer types across all treatment phases report elevations in many proinflammatory cytokines and markers of increased cytokine activity [2, 40-47]. For example, Kaminska et. al. [48] examined patients with diagnosed non-small cell lung cancer that did not receive treatment during a 6-year follow-up period and reported that TNF- α, IL-6, IL-8, soluble TNF receptor 1 (sTNFr1), sTNF-r2, soluble IL-2 receptor-alpha, IL-1receptor antagonist (IL-1ra) and IL-10 were significantly elevated compared with healthy controls. Furthermore, IL-10 levels were related to the tumour size and IL-6 levels were related to both tumour size and disease progression. Additionally, Pusztai et al. [49] examined breast cancer patients with and without primary tumour removal (neoadjuvant treatment vs. adjuvant treatment) receiving either low-dose paclitaxel chemotherapy treatments at one-week intervals (80mg/m^2 3-hr continuous infusion) or high-dose paclitaxel treatments at three-week intervals (175-225mg/m^2 24-h continuous infusion) and healthy controls and reported increased concentrations of IL-6 and IL-8 in the high-dose treatment group and an increased plasma concentration of IL-10 in the low-dose treatment group compared with healthy controls.

Additionally, the changes in proinflammatory cytokine levels observed were not different between the neoadjuvant or adjuvant treatments groups. Similar findings of elevated proinflammatory cytokine levels and markers of cytokine activity following radiation treatment have been reported in prostate cancer patients [50]. Together, these results demonstrate that cancer and its treatment are associated with elevated levels of proinflammatory cytokines and increased cytokine activity. Additionally, these results also indicate that the absence of treatment or the removal of the primary tumour prior to treatment may not alter the host inflammatory response. However, the specific proinflammatory response triggered may be mediated by the treatment regime received. Furthermore, elevations in proinflammatory cytokine levels and increased cytokine activity appear to be chronic consequences of cancer and its treatment and have been observed to persist in disease-free survivors for 5-10 years post-treatment [24].

Association between Cytokine Dysregulation and Cancer-related Fatigue

Despite the persistent increases in proinflammatory cytokine levels and markers of elevated cytokine activity associated with cancer and its treatment, relatively few studies have examined their relationship with CRF scores [51]. Panju et al. [52] reported in untreated patients with acute myeloid leukemia within 1 year of diagnosis that CRF was associated with IL-5, IL-6 and IL-10. These authors also reported that global quality of life was related to interferon-gamma, IL-2, IL-5, IL-8 and TNF-α. Greenberg et. al. [41] followed prostate cancer patients undergoing 8 weeks of localised radiation treatment and reported that weekly mean fatigue scores and IL-1 increased then plateaued by weeks 4 and 5, while fatigue scores further increased during weeks 6 and 7. Unfortunately, correlations between IL-1 and fatigue scores were not reported. More compelling data are provided by Wratten et al. [53] who followed breast cancer patients receiving radiotherapy and reported that fatigue scores were positively correlated with plasma levels of IL-6 and other markers of immune activity by week 4 of treatment, such as C-reactive protein, soluble thrombomodulin, tissue plasminogen activator, monocyte and neutrophil counts. Furthermore, Von Ah et al. [54] reported that IL-1β predicted CRF before adjuvant therapy in breast cancer patients. In contrast, however, other investigations have failed to observe increased proinflammatory cytokine levels despite significant fatigue in breast cancer patients receiving chest radiotherapy [55]], or correlations between fatigue scores and various proinflammatory cytokines or markers of inflammation in uterine cancer patients receiving radiation therapy [56] or in metastatic or locally advanced lung cancer patients receiving palliative care [57].

Studies examining the association between persistent fatigue and proinflammatory cytokines levels and markers of immune activity in long-term cancer survivors are also limited. Bower et al. [43] examined fatigued and non-fatigued disease-free breast cancer survivors 1-5 years post-diagnosis and reported that fatigued survivors had significantly higher plasma levels of IL-1ra, sTNF-r2, and neopterin than non-fatigued patients. Fatigued survivors also demonstrated a lower percentage of natural killer and naive (CD45RA+) CD4 T-cells, a higher percentage of memory (CD45RO+) CD4 T-cells, and a higher CD45RO+ to CD45RA+ CD4 T-cell ratio. Support for these findings are provided by Orre et al. [58] who examined testicular cancer survivors 11 years post-treatment and reported higher levels of IL-1ra and C-reactive protein in fatigued patients compared with non-fatigued patients. However, no differences were observed between groups in IL-6, sTNF-R1 or neopterin. Furthermore, it was observed using logical regression analyses that IL-1ra and C-reactive protein explained approximately 35% of the variance in CRF among patients. Collado-Hidaglo et al. [59] compared inflammatory and immune activity between fatigued and non-fatigued breast cancer survivors 2 years after successful primary therapy and reported that fatigued survivors were distinguishable from non-fatigued survivors by elevated levels of plasma IL-1ra and soluble IL-6r and decreased monocyte cell-surface IL-6 receptor (IL-6r) levels. Furthermore, fatigued survivors exhibited an exacerbated inflammatory response to lipopolysaccharide stimulation demonstrated by greater increases in IL-6 and TNF-α levels.

However, not all research findings are in agreement with these results. Gélinas and Fillion [60] examined post-treatment breast cancer survivors and did not observe an association between fatigue scores and IL-6. Other studies examining post-treatment hematological cancer patients also failed to observe associations between fatigue scores and markers of inflammation, such as plasma IL-1b, IL-1ra, IL-6, neopterin, CRP, and soluble TNF receptors [61, 62]. Discrepancies between studies examining the association between proinflammatory and immune activity markers and CRF may be explained by a number of reasons. Some studies in this area have used cross-sectional research designs and relatively small sample sizes, which may limit the ability to identify between group differences or relationships between variables within groups due to high data variance. Additionally, proinflammatory cytokine levels and markers of inflammation and immune activity have been reported to change through the course of treatment [50]. Thus, studies examining data collected at a single time point during a treatment cycle may not permit associations between variables to be observed [63]. Furthermore, because fatigue is a perceived phenomenon it can only be assessed using a subjective recall questionnaire that characterizes patient symptoms. In this regard, a number of questionnaires have been developed for this purpose, which has resulted in inconsistencies between studies in the methods used to assess fatigue status [22, 64-70]. Additionally, the psychometric properties of objective fatigue questionnaires and their clinical value in assessing fatigue status in cancer patients is debatable [10, 71]. Furthermore, similar to other subjective recall instruments, the results from cancer fatigue questionnaires may be influenced by self-reporting bias. As such, it has been suggested that as fatigue can persist for a prolonged period of time patients may experience a change in subjective standards of measurement throughout the course of the disease [72]. Thus, patients affected by prolonged CRF can gradually become accustomed to an impaired functonal status and experience it as normal [73]. This is supported by studies that fail to observe correlations between subjective fatigue scores and self-reported or objective physical activity levels [74] or measures of maximal physical performance despite significantly impaired physiological capacity [73-75].

Investigating Cancer-related Fatigue through Exercise-induced Fatigue

Much of what we know about the development of physical fatigue has come from research investigating exercise-induced fatigue. Research success in this area is largely due to the application of specialised electrophysiological and neurobiological assessment techniques that have allowed the physiological mechanisms contributing to exercise associated reductions in performance to be examined [76-83]. Based on the accumulation of data obtained the physiological mechanisms contributing to exercise-induced fatigue are broadly classified as either central or peripheral in origin [84]. Central fatigue occurs in the central nervous system (CNS) and is characterised by a progressive failure to voluntarily drive motor neurons causing a decline in motor unit recruitment and/or discharge frequency [25, 84], resulting from decreased excitability and/or inhibition of CNS, such as the motor cortex, descending upper motor axons, reflex inputs, or associated spinal circuitry. Peripheral fatigue occurs at the neuromuscular junction and/or within the muscle and is characterised by the inability of the peripheral contractile apparatus to perform work despite adequate central drive [25, 84]. Peripheral fatigue may occur due to neuromuscular transmission failure and/or a reduction in the function of the contractile apparatus as a result of reduced energy substrate availability and/or the accumulation of metabolic by-products.

Studies examining the central and peripheral contributions to exercise-induced changes in performance have been successfully performed in other pathologies that manifest as fatigue and have provided new insights into the pathophysiological mechanisms involved, such as chronic fatigue syndrome [85-89]. However, only one available study has examined CRF through exercise-induced fatigue. Yavuzsen et al. [30] compared the contributions of central and peripheral factors to exercise-induced fatigue between advanced cancer patients referred to palliative care and healthy controls. All subjects were assessed for fatigue using the Brief Fatigue Index questionnaire. Exercise testing involved participants sustaining a submaximal elbow flexion contraction at 30% maximal voluntary force until exhaustion. The authors reported that cancer patients had higher fatigue scores, a shorter time to exhaustion during the submaximal exercise task, and greater relative evoked twitch force following exercise compared with controls. Additionally, the relative loss in maximal voluntary force following the submaximal exercise task was lower in the cancer patients compared with controls. These data provide evidence to suggest that reduced sustained physical performance in the cancer patients was related to greater central fatigue. Such findings are consistent with results from studies examining exercise-induced fatigue in other neurological conditions [85-91]. However, the underlying pathophysiological mechanisms involved in the development of central fatigue in cancer and the association with cytokine dyregulation is unclear.

Potential Mechanisms by which Cytokine Dysregulation May Induce Central Fatigue in Cancer

Although the pathophysiology of CRF has not been clearly determined, a number of mechanisms involving cytokine dysregulation have been proposed to account for the variety of deleterious symptoms associated with cancer and its treatment [21, 23, 25, 27]. Such mechanisms typically include altered serotonin metabolism, hypothalamic-pituitary-adrenal axis (HPA) disruption and vagal afferent nerve activation. These mechanisms have been suggested as they are implicated in the pathophysiology of other chronic conditions that manifest as fatigue, such as chronic fatigue syndrome, rheumatoid arthritis and fibromyalgia [92, 93], the development of sickness-induced behaviours [34], and exercise-induced fatigue processes in healthy persons [78]. The following discussion outlines these mechanisms and describes the possible processes by which they may manifest in central fatigue in cancer. It must be noted that these mechanisms are likely to be interrelated and changes in the regulation of one mechanism may have downstream effects on the regulation of others. Furthermore, it is likely that the contribution of each of these mechanisms to CRF probably varies across time from initial diagnosis to long-term survival [23].

ALTERED SEROTONIN METABOLISM

Serotonin (5-HT) is a neurotransmitter that plays a critical role within the CNS regulating mood and behaviour. It has been proposed that the development of CRF may be related to increased brain 5-HT levels and/or the up-regulation of a population of 5-HT receptors contributing to reduced somatomotor drive, HPA axis distruption, and a sensation of a reduced capacity to perform physical work (Figure 1). Research examining exercise-induced fatigue and chronic fatigue syndrome provide evidence to suggest that altered 5-HT metabolism may play a role in the development of central fatigue. Because serotonin is unable to cross the blood-brain barrier, cerebral neurons are required to synthesis it locally from its peripheral precursor tryptophan [78]. As the enzyme that synthesises tryptophan into 5-HT is not saturated under normal conditions, the transport of tryptophan from the periphery through the blood-brain barrier is thought to be the rate limiting step in the central synthesis of 5-HT [94]. At rest, tryptophan competes with branched-chain amino acids (BCAA) for entry into the brain as they both share a common transporter system. However, during exercise BCAA are metabolised by skeletal muscle, allowing more tryptophan to enter the brain thus increasing the rate of 5-HT synthesis [95, 96]. Furthermore, increased concentrations of free-fatty acids associated with prolonged exercise may displace tryptophan from albumin in the blood, generating more free-tryptophan in the plasma available for 5-HT synthesis [78]. In this regard, some animal studies demonstrate that concentrations of 5-HT in the hypothalamus and brain stem increase with sustained exercise and the onset of fatigue is associated with peak 5-HT levels [97, 98] and elevated plasma levels of free tryptophan have been observed in chronic fatigue patients [91, 99, 100]. Furthermore, some studies [101, 102], but not all [103, 104], report that administering selective serotonin reuptake inhibitors prior to prolonged cycling exercise results in decreased exercise capacity in humans.

Experimental data demonstrate an association between proinflammatory cytokines and 5-HT metabolism. Clement et al. [105] examining rats observed that the acute administration of IL-1β and TNF-α intercerebroventrically or peripherally were associated with increases in extracellular levels of 5-HT and it's metabolite (5-HIAA) in the dorsal raphe nucleus, indicating an increase in 5-HT release into the synaptic space. Under normal conditions, a complex bi-directional relationship may exist where proinflammatory cytokines and 5-HT in the CNS regulate each other [106]. However, this feedback loop may become dysfunctional in cancer due to the greatly increased cytokine cascade. It is speculated that chronic elevations in proinflammatory cytokine levels may result in augmented and self-maintained levels of 5-HT transporter [27]. In this case, the brain may not synthesize adequate levels of 5-HT to overcome the increased transporter expression, which may result in altered serotoninergic neurotransmission and a greater propensity for central fatigue. Although some studies have reported that central 5-HT levels do not influence CRF [107, 108], these results may be biased based on the issues previously discussed regarding the limitations of using subjective questionnaires to assess CFR.

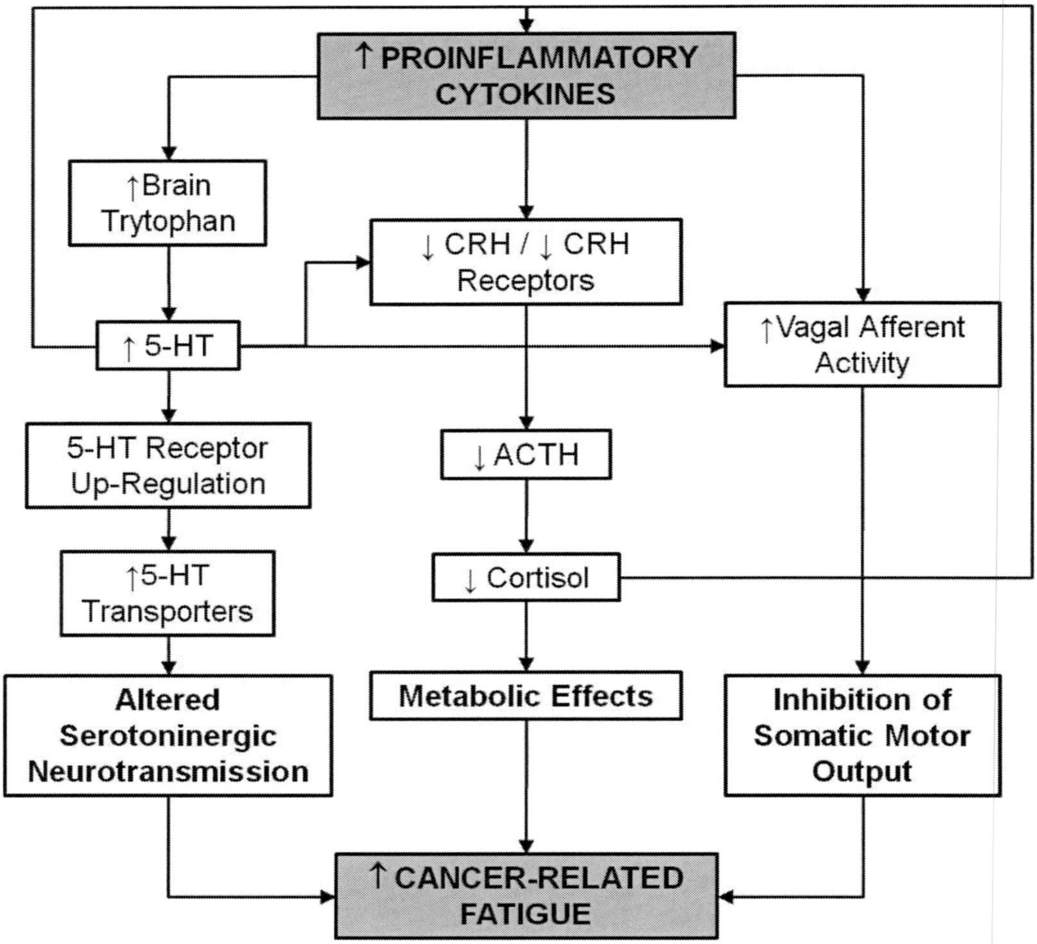

Figure 1. Schematic representation of the possible interactions between increased proinflammatory cytokine levels, altered serotonin metabolism, hypothalamus-pituitary-adrenal axis disruption and vagal afferent nerve activation and the development of cancer-related fatigue. 5-HT, serotonin; CRH, corticotropin-releasing hormone; ACTH, adrenocorticotropin hormone.

Hypothalamic-Pituitary-Adrenal Axis (HPA) Disruption

The HPA axis is the central endocrine system that regulates the release of the stress hormone cortisol [21]. The HPA axis disruption hypotheses suggests that cancer and its treatment directly or indirectly impairs HPA axis function resulting in reduced cortisol levels leading to the development of fatigue (Figure 1). Data obtained from healthy persons and clinical populations suggest hypocortisolemia may be involved in the aetiology of fatigue. Kumari et al. [109] reported that low waking salivary cortisol levels and a flat slope in diurnal cortisol secretion were associated with current and future fatigue scores in community dwelling adults. Additionally, the presence of hypocortisolemia is well documented in a variety of clinical conditions associated with fatigue, such as chronic fatigue syndrome [92] and fibromyalgia [110].

Lower waking cortisol levels [43] along with reduced function of the HPA axis demonstrated through a blunted cortisol stress response [111] are reported in fatigued breast cancer survivors with elevated proinflammatory cytokine levels. Furthermore, fatigued breast cancer survivors have a significantly flatter diurnal cortisol slope than non-fatigued survivors due to a less rapid decline in cortisol levels in the evening hours [112]. The use of certain cancer treatments has been observed to directly suppress HPA function and cortisol release. Radiation therapy and chemotherapy have been demonstrated to result in hypocortisolemia in children [113, 114]. Additionally, Del Priore et al. [115] assessed HPA function in patients receiving high-dose dexamethasone (DEX) as part of their chemotherapy regimen for epithelial ovarian cancer. HPA integrity was evaluated by administering synthetic adrenocorticotropic hormone (ACTH) and assessing cortisol levels 11-19 days after the completion of the DEX treatment. All patients demonstrated a sufficient increase in their plasma cortisol after ACTH stimulation, which suggests normal HPA function on the days tested. However, the increases in plasma cortisol at 30 and 60 min become lower as the interval from ACTH stimulation testing to the DEX regimen decreased. These data indicate that glucocorticoid prescribed with chemotherapy transiently decreases HPA function for approximately 8 days following treatment.

The mechanisms contributing to HPA axis disruption in cancer are not well known. However, it is now well established that communication between the CNS and the immune system is bidirectional in that endocrine changes can alter immune function and immune responses can alter both endocrine and CNS activity [116]. In this regard, studies examining animal models of chronic inflammatory conditions, such as adjuvant-induced arthritis, experimental allergic encephalomyelitis, exposure to parasites, report reductions in hypothalamic corticotrophin-releasing hormone (CRH) mRNA expression and that the HPA axis may be refractory to CRH during chronic stress [117-119]. In addition, down-regulation of the CRH receptors and reduced cortisol output may also be involved [120, 121]. However, it should be stated that the altered cortisol levels observed in cancer may be related to changes in circadian rhythm, rather than altered HPA axis function. Sleep disturbances and variations in rest–activity patterns are frequently reported by cancer patients and are independently associated with fatigue symptoms [122]. Furthermore, the mechanisms by which hypocortisolemia may induce fatigue in cancer are not known. It is well established that cortisol levels are regulated through a reciprocal interaction between 5-HT and the HPA axis as stimulation of 5-HT_{1A} [123] and 5-HT_{2C} [124] receptors signal the release of CRH and

ACTH. Therefore, under normal conditions elevated 5-HT should result in increased cortisol levels. The change in the relationship between 5-HT and cortisol levels associated with CRF warrants further investigation. Despite this, however, it is known that cortisol has an inhibitory effect on cytokine production [125]. As such, hypocortisolemia may result in increased plasma proinflammatory cytokine concentrations influencing 5-HT metabolism.

VAGAL AFFERENT NERVE ACTIVATION

The vagus nerve (cranial nerve X), consists of a large bundle of axons that transmit afferent signals from visceral organs to the brain stem and efferent parasympathetic signals from the brain stem to the viscera. The vagal afferent activation hypothesis proposes that the peripheral release of neuroactive substances associated with cancer and its treatment, such as 5-HT, proinflammatory cytokines and prostaglandins, may activate populations of vagal afferent fibres resulting in the reflex inhibition of somatic motor output [21, 25] (Figure 1). Schweitzer and Wright [126] document the presence of a vagosomatic inhibitory reflex reporting that electrical stimulation of the vagal afferent nerve resulted in a decrease in the amplitude of the tendon tap reflex in dogs. Since then, Ek et al. [127] have reported that in rats intravenously administered IL-1β increased the number of sensory neurons in the nodose ganglion expressing the cellular activation marker c-Fos coupled with increased discharge activity of vagal afferents arising from gastric compartments. However, this response was attenuated in animals pretreated with indomethacin, which inhibits prostaglandin production. These results suggest that afferent fibres of the vagus nerve express receptors to IL-1β and that circulating IL-1β and prostaglandins stimulate vagal afferent activity. Other animal studies demonstrate activation of populations of visceral afferent receptors in the thoracic cavity which inhibit somatic motor output or the stepping reflex in decerebrate and mesencephalic cats [128, 129] an rats [130]. Additionally, DiCarlo et al. [131] reported in rats that stimulation of vagal afferents using a 5-HT receptor during steady state exercise was associated with decreased muscle recruitment.

Although its presence in humans is yet to be observed [132, 133], a vagosomatic inhibitory reflex may account for the lethargy, muscle weakness, and greater perceived effort to complete a motor task that typically accompanies cancer and its treatment. The neuroactive substances previously described may be secreted in response to tumor growth or treatment in locations where vagal afferent fibres terminate and inhibit somatic motor activity. However, investigating the contribution of a vagosomatic inhibitory reflex to the development of central fatigue associated with cancer and its treatment would be challenging.

CONCLUSION

Considerable evidence exists demonstrating that cytokine dysregulation resulting from a chronic low grade inflammatory response is a significant consequence of cancer and its treatment and may contribute to the pathophysiological mechanisms involved in CRF. Although results from studies examining the association between cytokine dysregulation and CRF are conflicting, it is likely that such discrepancies are related to bias associated with the use of subjective recall questionnaires to assess fatigue status in cancer patients. Therefore, exercise-induced fatigue studies may provide new insight into CRF by examining the relationship between cytokine dysregulation and objective assessments of functional performance and fatigue status in cancer patients. Furthermore, such studies would allow the neurobiological mechanisms contributing to CRF to be examined, which would support or refute hypotheses for altered serotonin metabolism, HPA axis disruption, and/or vagal afferent nerve as pathophysiological mechanisms in the development of CRF.

REFERENCES

[1] Cella D, Peterman A, Passik S, Jacobsen P, Breitbart W. Progress toward guidelines for the management of fatigue. *Oncology,* 1998, 12, 369-77.

[2] Bower JE, Ganz PA, Desmond KA, Bernaards C, Rowland JH, Meyerowitz BE, et al. Fatigue in long-term breast carcinoma survivors. *Cancer*, 2006, 106, 751-8.

[3] Cella D, Davis K, Breitbart W, Curt G. Cancer-Related Fatigue: Prevalence of Proposed Diagnostic Criteria in a United States Sample of Cancer Survivors. *J Clin Oncol*, 2001, 19, 3385-91.

[4] Stone P, Richards M, A'Hern R, Hardy J. A study to investigate the prevalence, severity and correlates of fatigue among patients with cancer in comparison with a control group of volunteers without cancer. *Ann Oncol*, 2000, 11, 561-7.

[5] Vogelzang NJ, Breitbart W, Cella D, Curt GA, Groopman JE, Horning SJ, et al. Patient, caregiver, and oncologist perceptions of cancer-related fatigue: results of a tripart assessment survey. The Fatigue Coalition. *Semin Hematol*, 1997, 34, 4-12.

[6] Hickok JT, Morrow GR, Roscoe JA, Mustian K, Okunieff P. Occurrence, Severity, and Longitudinal Course of Twelve Common Symptoms in 1129 Consecutive Patients During Radiotherapy for Cancer. *J Pain Symptom Manage*, 2005, 30, 433-42.

[7] Stone P, Richardson A, Ream E, Smith AG, Kerr DJ, Kearney N, et al. Cancer-related fatigue: Inevitable, unimportant and untreatable? Results of a multi-centre patient survey. *Ann Oncol*, 2000, 11, 971-5.

[8] Holley S. Cancer-Related Fatigue. *Cancer Pract*, 2000, 8, 87-95.

[9] Curt GA, Breitbart W, Cella D, Groopman JE, Horning SJ, Itri LM, et al. Impact of Cancer-Related Fatigue on the Lives of Patients: New Findings From the Fatigue Coalition. *Oncologist*, 2000, 5, 353-60.

[10] Wu H-S, McSweeney M. Cancer-related fatigue: "It's so much more than just being tired". *Eur J Oncol Nurs*, 2007, 11, 117-25.

[11] Díaz N, Menjón S, Rolfo C, García-Alonso P, Carulla J, Magro A, et al. Patients' perception of cancer-related fatigue: results of a survey to assess the impact on their everyday life. *Clin Transl Oncol*, 2008, 10, 753-7.

[12] van den Beuken-van Everdingen MHJ, de Rijke J, M., Kessels AG, Schouten HC, van Kleef M, Patijn J. Quality of Life and Non-Pain Symptoms in Patients with Cancer. *J Pain Symptom Manage*, 2009, 38, 216-33.

[13] Hofman M, Ryan JL, Figueroa-Moseley CD, Jean-Pierre P, Morrow GR. Cancer-Related Fatigue: The Scale of the Problem. *Oncologist*, 2007, 12, 4-10.

[14] Lawrence DP, Kupelnick B, Miller K, Devine D, Lau J. Evidence report on the occurrence, assessment, and treatment of fatigue in cancer patients. *J Natl Cancer Inst Monogr*, 2004, 40-50.

[15] Jacobsen PB, Hann DM, Azzarello LM, Horton J, Balducci L, Lyman GH. Fatigue in Women Receiving Adjuvant Chemotherapy for Breast Cancer: Characteristics, Course, and Correlates. *J Pain Symptom Manage*, 1999, 18, 233-42.

[16] Forlenza MJ, Hall P, Lichtenstein P, Evengard B, Sullivan PF. Epidemiology of cancer-related fatigue in the Swedish twin registry. *Cancer*, 2005, 104, 2022-31.

[17] Latvala A, Syrjanen K, Salmenoja H, Salminen E. Anaemia and other predictors of fatigue among patients on palliative therapy for advanced cancer. *Anticancer Res*, 2009, 29, 2569-75.

[18] Brintzenhofe-Szoc KM, Levin TT, Li Y, Kissane DW, Zabora JR. Mixed Anxiety/Depression Symptoms in a Large Cancer Cohort: Prevalence by Cancer Type. *Psychosomatics*, 2009, 50, 383-91.

[19] Craig TJ, Abeloff MD. Psychiatric symptomatology among hospitalized cancer patients. *Am J Psychiatry*, 1974, 131, 1323-7.

[20] Ancoli-Israel S, Moore PJ, Jones V. The relationship between fatigue and sleep in cancer patients: a review. *Eur J Cancer Care (Engl)*, 2001, 10, 245-55.

[21] Wang XS. Pathophysiology of Cancer-Related Fatigue. *Clin J Oncol Nurs*, 2008, 12, 11-20.

[22] Mendoza TR, Wang XS, Cleeland CS, Morrissey M, Johnson BA, Wendt JK, et al. The rapid assessment of fatigue severity in cancer patients: use of the Brief Fatigue Inventory. *Cancer*, 1999, 85, 1186-96.

[23] Cheville AL. Cancer-Related Fatigue. *Phys Med Rehabil Clin N Am*, 2009, 20, 405-16.

[24] Bower JE. Cancer-related fatigue: links with inflammation in cancer patients and survivors. *Brain Behav Immun*, 2007, 21, 863-71.

[25] Ryan JL, Carroll JK, Ryan EP, Mustian KM, Fiscella K, Morrow GR. Mechanisms of Cancer-Related Fatigue. *Oncologist*, 2007, 12, 22-34.

[26] Kurzrock R. The role of cytokines in cancer-related fatigue. *Cancer*, 2001, 92, 1684-8.

[27] Morrow G, Andrews P, Hickok J, Roscoe J, Matteson S. Fatigue associated with cancer and its treatment. *Support Care Cancer*, 2002, 10, 389-98.

[28] Levy MR. Cancer Fatigue: A Neurobiological Review for Psychiatrists. *Psychosomatics*, 2008, 49, 283-91.

[29] Wood L, Nail L, Gilster A, Winters K, Elsea C. Cancer Chemotherapy-Related Symptoms: Evidence to Suggest a Role for Proinflammatory Cytokines. *Oncol Nurs Forum*, 2006, 33, 535-42.

[30] Yavuzsen T, Davis MP, Ranganathan VK, Walsh D, Siemionow V, Kirkova J, et al. Cancer-Related Fatigue: Central or Peripheral? *J Pain Symptom Manage*, In press, EPub online first.

[31] Myers J. Proinflammatory Cytokines and Sickness Behavior: Implications for Depression and Cancer-Related Symptoms. *Oncol Nurs Forum*, 2008, 35, 802-7.

[32] Borish L, Schmaling K, DiClementi JD, Streib J, Negri J, Jones JF. Chronic fatigue syndrome: identification of distinct subgroups on the basis of allergy and psychologic variables. *J Allergy Clin Immunol*, 1998, 102, 222-30.

[33] Blesch KS, Paice JA, Wickham R, Harte N, Schnoor DK, Purl S, et al. Correlates of fatigue in people with breast or lung cancer. *Oncol Nurs Forum*, 1991, 18, 81-7.

[34] Dantzer R. Cytokine-Induced Sickness Behavior: Mechanisms and Implications. *Ann N Y Acad Sci*, 2001, 933, 222-34.
[35] Malik UR, Makower DF, Wadler S. Interferon-mediated fatigue. *Cancer*, 2001, 92, 1664-8.
[36] Connor TJ, O'Sullivan J, Nolan Y, Kelly JP. Inhibition of constitutive nitric oxide production increases the severity of lipopolysaccharide-induced sickness behaviour: a role for TNF-alpha. *Neuroimmunomodulation*, 2002, 10, 367-78.
[37] Bluthe RM, Walter V, Parnet P, Laye S, Lestage J, Verrier D, et al. Lipopolysaccharide induces sickness behaviour in rats by a vagal mediated mechanism. *C R Acad Sci III*, 1994, 317, 499-503.
[38] Rakoff-Nahoum S. Why cancer and inflammation? *Yale J Biol Med*, 2006, 79, 123-30.
[39] Aggarwal BB, Vijayalekshmi RV, Sung B. Targeting inflammatory pathways for prevention and therapy of cancer: short-term friend, long-term foe. *Clin Cancer Res*, 2009, 15, 425-30.
[40] Bianco JA, Appelbaum FR, Nemunaitis J, Almgren J, Andrews F, Kettner P, et al. Phase I-II trial of pentoxifylline for the prevention of transplant- related toxicities following bone marrow transplantation. *Blood*, 1991, 78, 1205-11.
[41] Greenberg DB, Gray JL, Mannix CM, Eisenthal S, Carey M. Treatment-related fatigue and serum interleukin-1 levels in patients during external beam irradiation for prostate cancer. *J Pain Symptom Manage*, 1993, 8, 196-200.
[42] Hong J-H, Chiang C-S, Campbell IL, Sun J-R, Withers HR, McBride WH. Induction of acute phase gene expression by brain irradiation. *Int J Rad Oncol Biol Phys*, 1995, 33, 619-26.
[43] Bower JE, Ganz PA, Aziz N, Fahey JL. Fatigue and Proinflammatory Cytokine Activity in Breast Cancer Survivors. *Psychosom Med*, 2002, 64, 604-11.
[44] Ikeguchi M, Hatada T, Yamamoto M, Miyake T, Matsunaga T, Fukumoto Y, et al. Serum interleukin-6 and -10 levels in patients with gastric cancer. *Gastric Cancer*, 2009, 12, 95-100.
[45] Rutkowski P, Kami J, nacute, ska, Kowalska M, Ruka W, et al. Cytokine and cytokine receptor serum levels in adult bone sarcoma patients: Correlations with local tumor extent and prognosis. *J Surg Oncol*, 2003, 84, 151-9.
[46] Kaminska J, Kowalska MM, Nowacki MP, Chwalinski MG, Rysinska A, Fuksiewicz M. CRP, TNF-alpha, IL-1ra, IL-6, IL-8 and IL-10 in blood serum of colorectal cancer patients. *Pathol Oncol Res*, 2000, 6, 38-41.
[47] Rutkowski P, Kaminska J, Kowalska M, Ruka W, Steffen J. Cytokine serum levels in soft tissue sarcoma patients: Correlations with clinico-pathological features and prognosis. *Int J Cancer*, 2002, 100, 463-71.
[48] Kaminska J, Kowalska M, Kotowicz B, Fuksiewicz M, Glogowski M, Wojcik E, et al. Pretreatment serum levels of cytokines and cytokine receptors in patients with non-small cell lung cancer, and correlations with clinicopathological features and prognosis. M-CSF - an independent prognostic factor. *Oncology*, 2006, 70, 115-25.
[49] Pusztai L, Mendoza TR, Reuben JM, Martinez MM, Willey JS, Lara J, et al. Changes in plasma levels of inflammatory cytokines in response to paclitaxel chemotherapy. *Cytokine*, 2004, 25, 94-102.

[50] Bower JE, Ganz PA, Tao ML, Hu W, Belin TR, Sepah S, et al. Inflammatory biomarkers and fatigue during radiation therapy for breast and prostate cancer. *Clin Cancer Res*, 2009, 15, 5534-40.

[51] Schubert C, Hong S, Natarajan L, Mills PJ, Dimsdale JE. The association between fatigue and inflammatory marker levels in cancer patients: a quantitative review. *Brain Behav Immun*, 2007, 21, 413-27.

[52] Panju AH, Danesh A, Minden MD, Kelvin DJ, Alibhai SM. Associations between quality of life, fatigue, and cytokine levels in patients aged 50+ with acute myeloid leukemia. *Suppt Care Canc*, 2009, 17, 539-46.

[53] Wratten C, Kilmurray J, Nash S, Seldon M, Hamilton CS, O'Brien PC, et al. Fatigue during breast radiotherapy and its relationship to biological factors. *Int J Radiat Oncol Biol Phys*, 2004, 59, 160-7.

[54] Von Ah DM, Kang DH, Carpenter JS. Predictors of cancer-related fatigue in women with breast cancer before, during, and after adjuvant therapy. *Cancer Nurs*, 2008, 31, 134-44.

[55] Geinitz H, Zimmermann FB, Stoll P, Thamm R, Kaffenberger W, Ansorg K, et al. Fatigue, serum cytokine levels, and blood cell counts during radiotherapy of patients with breast cancer. *Int J Radiat Oncol Biol Phys*, 2001, 51, 691-8.

[56] Ahlberg K, Ekman T, Gaston-Johansson F. Levels of Fatigue Compared to Levels of Cytokines and Hemoglobin during Pelvic Radiotherapy: a Pilot Study. *Biol Res Nurs*, 2004, 5, 203-10.

[57] Brown DJF, McMillan DC, Milroy R. The correlation between fatigue, physical function, the systemic inflammatory response, and psychological distress in patients with advanced lung cancer. *Cancer*, 2005, 103, 377-82.

[58] Orre IJ, Murison R, Dahl AA, Ueland T, Aukrust P, Fossa SD. Levels of circulating interleukin-1 receptor antagonist and C-reactive protein in long-term survivors of testicular cancer with chronic cancer-related fatigue. *Brain Behav Immun*, 2009, 23, 868-74.

[59] Collado-Hidalgo A, Bower JE, Ganz PA, Cole SW, Irwin MR. Inflammatory biomarkers for persistent fatigue in breast cancer survivors. *Clin Cancer Res*, 2006, 12, 2759-66.

[60] Gélinas C, Fillion L. Factors Related to Persistent Fatigue Following Completion of Breast Cancer Treatment. *Oncol Nurs Forum*, 2004, 31, 269-78.

[61] Dimeo F, Schmittel A, Fietz T, Schwartz S, Kohler P, Boning D, et al. Physical performance, depression, immune status and fatigue in patients with hematological malignancies after treatment. *Ann Oncol*, 2004, 15, 1237-42.

[62] Knobel H, Loge JH, Nordoy T, Kolstad AL, Espevik T, Kvaloy S, et al. High level of fatigue in lymphoma patients treated with high dose therapy. *J Pain Symp Manag*, 2000, 19, 446-56.

[63] Quatan N, Meyer B, Bailey M, Pandha H. Persistently high levels of immunosuppressive cytokines in patients after radical prostatectomy. *Prostate Canc Prost Dis*, 2006, 9, 420-5.

[64] Jacobsen PB. Assessment of Fatigue in Cancer Patients. *J Natl Cancer Inst Monogr*, 2004, 2004, 93-7.

[65] Piper BF, Dibble SL, Dodd MJ, Weiss MC, Slaughter RE, Paul SM. The revised Piper Fatigue Scale: psychometric evaluation in women with breast cancer. *Oncol Nurs Forum*, 1998, 25, 677-84.

[66] Okuyama T, Tatsuo. A, Kugaya A, Okamura H, Shima Y, Maruguchi M, et al. Development and Validation of the Cancer Fatigue Scale: A Brief, Three-Dimensional, Self-Rating Scale for Assessment of Fatigue in Cancer Patients. *J Pain Symp Manag*, 2000, 19, 5-14.

[67] Schwartz A, Meek P. Additional construct validity of the Schwartz Cancer Fatigue Scale. *J Nurs Meas*, 1999, 7, 35-45.

[68] Smets EM, Garssen B, Bonke B, De Haes JC. The Multidimensional Fatigue Inventory (MFI) psychometric qualities of an instrument to assess fatigue. *J Psychosom Res*, 1995, 39, 315-25.

[69] Stein KD, Martin SC, Hann DM, Jacobsen PB. A Multidimensional Measure of Fatigue for Use with Cancer Patients. *Cancer Pract*, 1998, 6, 143-52.

[70] Yellen SB, Cella DF, Webster K, Blendowski C, Kaplan E. Measuring fatigue and other anemia-related symptoms with the Functional Assessment of Cancer Therapy (FACT) measurement system. *J Pain Symp Manag*, 1997, 13, 63-74.

[71] Wu HS, McSweeney M. Measurement of fatigue in people with cancer. *Oncol Nurs Forum*, 2001, 28, 1371-84; quiz 85-6.

[72] Breetvelt IS, Van Dam FS. Underreporting by cancer patients: the case of response-shift. *Soc Sci Med*, 1991, 32, 981-7.

[73] Dimeo F, Stieglitz R-D, Novelli-Fischer U, Fetscher S, Mertelsmann R, Keul J. Correlation between physical performance and fatigue in cancer patients. *Ann Oncol*, 1997, 8, 1251-5.

[74] Servaes P, Verhagen CAHHVM, Bleijenberg G. Relations between fatigue, neuropsychological functioning, and physical activity after treatment for breast carcinoma. *Cancer*, 2002, 95, 2017-26.

[75] Young KE, White CA. The prevalence and moderators of fatigue in people who have been successfully treated for cancer. *J Psychosom Res*, 2006, 60, 29-38.

[76] Herbert RD, Gandevia SC. Twitch interpolation in human muscles: Mechanisms and implications for measurement of voluntary activation. *J Neurophysiol*, 1999, 82, 2271-83.

[77] Shield A, Zhou S. Assessing voluntary muscle activation with the twitch interpolation technique. *Sports Med*, 2004, 34, 253-67.

[78] Meeusen R, Watson P, Hasegawa H, Roelands B, Piacentini MF. Central Fatigue: The Serotonin Hypothesis and Beyond. *Sports Med*, 2006, 36, 881-909.

[79] Racinais S, Girard O, Micallef JP, Perrey S. Failed excitability of spinal motoneurons induced by prolonged running exercise. *J Neurophysiol*, 2007, 97, 596-603.

[80] Sacco P, Thickbroom GW, Byrnes ML, Mastiaglia FL. Changes in corticomotor excitability after fatiguing muscle contractions. *Muscle Nerve*, 2000, 23, 1840-6.

[81] Meeusen R, Watson P, Hasegawa H, Roelands B, Piacentini MF. Brain neurotransmitters in fatigue and overtraining. *Appl Physiol Nutr Metab*, 2007, 32, 857-64.

[82] Ross EZ, Middleton N, Shave R, George K, Nowicky A. Human, Environmental & Exercise: Corticomotor excitability contributes to neuromuscular fatigue following marathon running in man. *Exp Physiol*, 2007, 92, 417-26.

[83] Foley T, Fleshner M. Neuroplasticity of Dopamine Circuits After Exercise: Implications for Central Fatigue. *Neuromolecular Med*, 2008, 10, 67-80.
[84] Gandevia SC. Spinal and Supraspinal Factors in Human Muscle Fatigue. *Physiol Rev*, 2001, 81, 1725-89.
[85] Samii A, Wassermann EM, Ikoma K, Mercuri B, George MS, O'Fallon A, et al. Decreased postexercise facilitation of motor evoked potentials in patients with chronic fatigue syndrome or depression. *Neurology*, 1996, 47, 1410-4.
[86] Sacco P, Hope PAJ, Thickbroom GW, Byrnes ML, Mastaglia FL. Corticomotor excitability and perception of effort during sustained exercise in the chronic fatigue syndrome. *Clinical Neurophysiol*, 1999, 110, 1883-91.
[87] Siemionow V, Fang Y, Calabrese L, Sahgal V, Yue GH. Altered central nervous system signal during motor performance in chronic fatigue syndrome. *Clin Neurophysiol*, 2004, 115, 2372-81.
[88] Schillings ML, Kalkman JS, Werf SPvd, Engelen BGMv, Bleijenberg G, Zwarts MJ. Diminished central activation during maximal voluntary contraction in chronic fatigue syndrome. *Clinical Neurophysiology*, 2004, 115, 2518-24.
[89] Chen R, Liang FX, Moriya J, Yamakawa J, Sumino H, Kanda T, et al. Chronic fatigue syndrome and the central nervous system. *J Int Med Res*, 2008, 36, 867-74.
[90] Chaudhuri A, Behan PO. Fatigue in neurological disorders. *Lancet*, 2004, 363, 978-88.
[91] Georgiades E, Behan WMH, Kilduff LP, Hadjicharalambous M, Mackie EE, Wilson J, et al. Chronic fatigue syndrome: new evidence for a central fatigue disorder. *Clin Sci*, 2003, 105, 213-8.
[92] Cleare AJ. The Neuroendocrinology of Chronic Fatigue Syndrome. *Endocr Rev*, 2003, 24, 236-52.
[93] Parker AJ, Wessely S, Cleare AJ. The neuroendocrinology of chronic fatigue syndrome and fibromyalgia. *Psychol Med*, 2001, 31, 1331-45.
[94] Fernstrom JD. Role of precursor availability in control of monoamine biosynthesis in brain. *Physiol Rev*, 1983, 63, 484-546.
[95] Newsholme EA, Blomstrand E. Branched-Chain Amino Acids and Central Fatigue. *J Nutr*, 2006, 136, 274S-6.
[96] Blomstrand E. A Role for Branched-Chain Amino Acids in Reducing Central Fatigue. *J Nutr*, 2006, 136, 544S-7.
[97] Bailey SP, Davis JM, Ahlborn EN. Neuroendocrine and substrate responses to altered brain 5-HT activity during prolonged exercise to fatigue. *J Appl Physiol*, 1993, 74, 3006-12.
[98] Blomstrand E, Perrett D, Parry-Billings M, Newsholme EA. Effect of sustained exercise on plasma amino acid concentrations and on 5-hydroxytryptamine metabolism in six different brain regions in the rat. *Acta Physiol Scand*, 1989, 136, 473-81.
[99] Fernstrom JD, Fernstrom MH. Exercise, serum free tryptophan, and central fatigue. *J Nutr*, 2006, 136, 553S-9S.
[100] Castell LM, Yamamoto T, Phoenix J, Newsholme EA. The role of tryptophan in fatigue in different conditions of stress. *Adv Exp Med Biol*, 1999, 467, 697-704.
[101] Wilson W, Maughan R. Evidence for a possible role of 5-hydroxytryptamine in the genesis of fatigue in man: administration of paroxetine, a 5-HT re-uptake inhibitor, reduces the capacity to perform prolonged exercise. *Exp Physiol*, 1992, 77, 921-4.

[102] Struder HK, Hollmann W, Platen P, Donike M, Gotzmann A, Weber K. Influence of paroxetine, branched-chain amino acids and tyrosine on neuroendocrine system responses and fatigue in humans. *Horm Metab Res*, 1998, 30, 188-94.

[103] Parise G, Bosman MJ, Boecker DR, Barry MJ, Tarnopolsky MA. Selective serotonin reuptake inhibitors: Their effect on high-intensity exercise performance. *Arch Phys Med Rehabil*, 2001, 82, 867-71.

[104] Meeusen R, Piacentini MF, Van Den Eynde S, Magnus L, De Meirleir K. Exercise performance is not influenced by a 5-HT reuptake inhibitor. *Int J Sports Med*, 2001, 22, 329-36.

[105] Clement HW, Buschmann J, Rex S, Grote C, Opper C, Gemsa D, et al. Effects of interferon-γ, interleukin-1β, and tumor necrosis factor-α on the serotonin metabolism in the nucleus raphe dorsalis of the rat. *J Neural Transm*, 1997, 104, 981-91.

[106] Pauli S, Linthorst ACE, Reul JMHM. Tumour necrosis factor-alpha and interleukin-2 differentially affect hippocampal serotonergic neurotransmission, behavioural activity, body temperature and hypothalamic-pituitary-adrenocortical axis activity in the rat. *Eur J Neurosci*, 1998, 10, 868-78.

[107] Morrow GR, Hickok JT, Roscoe JA, Raubertas RF, Andrews PLR, Flynn PJ, et al. Differential Effects of Paroxetine on Fatigue and Depression: A Randomized, Double-Blind Trial From the University of Rochester Cancer Center Community Clinical Oncology Program. *J Clin Oncol*, 2003, 21, 4635-41.

[108] Roscoe J, Morrow G, Hickok J, Mustian K, Griggs J, Matteson S, et al. Effect of paroxetine hydrochloride (Paxil®) on fatigue and depression in breast cancer patients receiving chemotherapy. *Breast Cancer Res Treat*, 2005, 89, 243-9.

[109] Kumari M, Badrick E, Chandola T, Adam EK, Stafford M, Marmot MG, et al. Cortisol secretion and fatigue: Associations in a community based cohort. *Psychoneuro endocrinol*, 2009.

[110] Izquierdo-Alvarez S, Bocos-Terraz J, Bancalero-Flores J, Pavon-Romero L, Serrano-Ostariz E, de Miquel C. Is there an association between fibromyalgia and below-normal levels of urinary cortisol? *BMC Research Notes*, 2008, 1, 134.

[111] Bower JE, Ganz PA, Aziz N. Altered Cortisol Response to Psychologic Stress in Breast Cancer Survivors With Persistent Fatigue. *Psychosom Med*, 2005, 67, 277-80.

[112] Bower JE, Ganz PA, Dickerson SS, Petersen L, Aziz N, Fahey JL. Diurnal cortisol rhythm and fatigue in breast cancer survivors. *Psychoneuroendocrinol*, 2005, 30, 92-100.

[113] Schmiegelow M, Feldt-Rasmussen U, Rasmussen AK, Lange M, Poulsen HS, Muller J. Assessment of the Hypothalamo-Pituitary-Adrenal Axis in Patients Treated with Radiotherapy and Chemotherapy for Childhood Brain Tumor. *J Clin Endocrinol Metab*, 2003, 88, 3149-54.

[114] Oberfield SE, Nirenberg A, Allen JC, Cohen H, Donahue B, Prasad V, et al. Hypothalamic-pituitary-adrenal function following cranial irradiation. *Horm Res*, 1997, 47, 9-16.

[115] Del Priore G, Gurski KJ, Warshal DP, Angel C, Dubeshter B. Adrenal function following high-dose steroids in ovarian cancer patients. *Gynecol Oncol*, 1995, 59, 102-4.

[116] Shanks N, Harbuz MS, Jessop DS, Perks P, Moore PM, Lightman SL. Inflammatory disease as chronic stress. *Ann N Y Acad Sci*, 1998, 840, 599-607.

[117] Harbuz MS, Leonard JP, Lightman SL, Cuzner ML. Changes in hypothalamic corticotrophin-releasing factor and anterior pituitary pro-opiomelanocortin mRNA during the course of experimental allergic encephalomyelitis. *J Neuroimmunol*, 1993, 45, 127-32.

[118] Harbuz MS, Rees RG, Eckland D, Jessop DS, Brewerton D, Lightman SL. Paradoxical responses of hypothalamic corticotropin-releasing factor (CRF) messenger ribonucleic acid (mRNA) and CRF-41 peptide and adenohypophysial proopiomelanocortin mRNA during chronic inflammatory stress. *Endocrinol*, 1992, 130, 1394-400.

[119] Whitnall MH. Regulation of the hypothalamic corticotropin-releasing hormone neurosecretory system. *Prog Neurobiol*, 1993, 40, 573-629.

[120] Cleare AJ, Miell J, Heap E, Sookdeo S, Young L, Malhi GS, et al. Hypothalamo-pituitary-adrenal axis dysfunction in chronic fatigue syndrome, and the effects of low-dose hydrocortisone therapy. *J Clin Endocrinol Metab*, 2001, 86, 3545-54.

[121] Demitrack MA, Dale JK, Straus SE, Laue L, Listwak SJ, Kruesi MJ, et al. Evidence for impaired activation of the hypothalamic-pituitary-adrenal axis in patients with chronic fatigue syndrome. *J Clin Endocrinol Metab*, 1991, 73, 1224-34.

[122] Roscoe JA, Kaufman ME, Matteson-Rusby SE, Palesh OG, Ryan JL, Kohli S, et al. Cancer-Related Fatigue and Sleep Disorders. *Oncologist*, 2007, 12, 35-42.

[123] Chaouloff F. Physiopharmacological interactions between stress hormones and central serotonergic systems. *Brain Res Brain Res Rev*, 1993, 18, 1-32.

[124] Heisler LK, Pronchuk N, Nonogaki K, Zhou L, Raber J, Tung L, et al. Serotonin Activates the Hypothalamic-Pituitary-Adrenal Axis via Serotonin 2C Receptor Stimulation. *J Neurosci*, 2007, 27, 6956-64.

[125] Petrovsky N, McNair P, Harrison LC. Diurnal rhythms of pro-inflammatory cytokines: regulation by plasma cortisol and therapeutic implications. *Cytokine*, 1998, 10, 307-12.

[126] Schweitzer A, Wright S. The anti-strychnine action of acetylcholine, prostigmine and related substances, and of central vagus stimulation. *J Physiol*, 1937, 90, 310-29.

[127] Ek M, Kurosawa M, Lundeberg T, Ericsson A. Activation of Vagal Afferents after Intravenous Injection of Interleukin-1beta : Role of Endogenous Prostaglandins. *J Neurosci*, 1998, 18, 9471-9.

[128] Anand A, Paintal AS. Reflex effects following selective stimulation of J receptors in the cat. *J Physiol*, 1980, 299, 553-72.

[129] Pickar JG, Hill JM, Kaufman MP. Stimulation of vagal afferents inhibits locomotion in mesencephalic cats. *J Appl Physiol*, 1993, 74, 103-10.

[130] Kawasaki K, Kodama M, Matsushita A. Caerulein, a cholecystokinin-related peptide, depresses somatic function via the vagal afferent system. *Life Sci*, 1983, 33, 1045-50.

[131] DiCarlo SE, Collins HL, Chen CY. Vagal afferents reflexly inhibit exercise in conscious rats. *Med Sci Sports Exerc*, 1994, 26, 459-62.

[132] Gandevia SC, Butler JE, Taylor JL, Crawford MR. Absence of viscerosomatic inhibition with injections of lobeline designed to activate human pulmonary C fibres. *J Physiol*, 1998, 511, 289-300.

[133] Widdicombe JG. The J Reflex. *J Physiol*, 1998, 511, 2.

In: Regulation of Fatigue in Exercise
Editor: Frank E. Marino

ISBN 978-1-61209-334-5

Chapter 9

AN OVERVIEW OF THE EPIDEMIOLOGICAL EVIDENCE LINKING INJURY RISK TO FATIGUE IN SPORT: IDENTIFICATION OF RESEARCH NEEDS AND OPPORTUNITIES

Caroline F. Finch[1*], Ann Williamson[2] and Brendan O'Brien[3]
[1]Australian Centre for Research into Injury in Sport and its Prevention (ACRISP) Monash, Injury Research Institute, Monash University, Clayton, Victoria, Australia
[2]School of Aviation, University of New South Wales, NSW, Australia
[3]School of Human Movement and Sport Sciences, University of Ballarat, Mt Helen, Victoria, Australia

ABSTRACT

Despite the large literature on the role of fatigue and injury risk in road and occupational settings, evidence for a direct causal link between sports injury risk and fatigue has not previously been reported. This Chapter summarises the epidemiological evidence linking fatigue to sport injury risk, identifies gaps in knowledge relating fatigue and sport injury risk and examines the potential for translating fatigue research from other injury contexts as a means of improving the knowledge base with regards to sports injury. Drawing on the broader fatigue and injury literature linking injury risk to fatigue, fatigue can potentially impact on sport performance/injury risk in one of two ways (or a combination of both): from a cognitive or central fatigue view or through musculoskeletal fatigue. In terms of cognitive-related fatigue, the likely contributors are: 1) sleep homeostasis factors including how long since slept, length of sleep period, quality of recent sleep; 2) circadian or time-of-day factors; and 3) task-related factors (e.g. level of activity) inherent in sport. In terms of musculoskeletal fatigue, physiological factors appear to be mainly associated with inhibited motor control and failure of the brakes of excessive tension development within muscles.

* E-mail: caroline.finch@monash.edu

This Chapter highlights the lack of epidemiological studies directly linking fatigue to injury risk and where they exist, the poor conceptualisation and measurement of fatigue which limits conclusions. Most of the published studies in this area are related to football codes: rugby (league or union) or soccer. Fatigue is generally identified in these studies in terms of associations between observed injury incidence patterns and the phase-of-play or time-of-season when the injury occurred. Most importantly, whilst the epidemiological studies may conclude that fatigue is a likely or possible risk factor for injury, no prospective study has yet attempted to formally measure fatigue and directly relate it to injury incidence. Overall, this Chapter highlights a need for further epidemiological research on the role of fatigue in sports injury. In lieu of direct evidence, the Chapter reviews the physiological basis for a link between fatigue and musculoskeletal injury risk and discusses the evidence for effects of "cognitive" fatigue on sports performance that is likely to raise injury risk. The Chapter then combines this fundamental evidence for fatigue effects with aetiological models for sports injury causation to highlight key areas where significant knowledge gaps currently exist. Finally, suggestions for a future research agenda that adopts a truly multidisciplinary research strategy are given, for this very important topic.

INTRODUCTION

There is strong accumulated evidence that fatigue plays a key role in the causes of injuries that occur in settings such as workplaces and on-the-road [1, 2]. More recently, it has been suggested that fatigue also plays a role in the aetiology of musculoskeletal injuries, such as those sustained by athletes and other sports participants, although no strong long-term prospective studies have yet confirmed this. Most formal evidence of a link between fatigue and sports injury comes from experimental studies or extrapolation of animal study results and fundamental biomechanics. The much larger body of indirect evidence comes from observational studies conducted largely in team sports.

A systematic review process was undertaken to identify peer-review literature published from 1990-2009, inclusive through an extensive electronic database search and hand searching of tables of contents for 2000-2009 for selected relevant journals. Keywords used in the search related to sport injury and sport injury risk, together with synonyms of physical fatigue (i.e. fatigue, overload, exhaustion, accumulation, lethargy, tiredness), time of play (i.e. phase, stage, quarter, period, half, season, session) and type of play (i.e., game, event, race, tournament, competition, match, meet). Whilst lab-based, clinical-based and field-based experimental studies were initially included as part of the background material search to justify a link between injury risk and fatigue, they were excluded in the final review presented here which focuses solely on epidemiological studies. To be included, studies needed to have monitored players or athletes during sporting events, conducted some form of injury surveillance and reporting and to have a focus on injury incidence, not adverse outcomes following injury (such as poor recovery). From an initial 457 original research articles relating to some aspect of fatigue in sport, only 61 were found to meet the above definition of an epidemiological study.

Table 1 summarizes the types of sports and their particular characteristics that have been most commonly reported to be associated with high levels of fatigue and, often inferred, corresponding injury risk.

Table 1. The sports most commonly linked to fatigue and associated increased injury risk

Type of sport and sport/characteristics [refs]	Illustrative examples of links between fatigue and injury in these sports [refs]
Endurance sports participated in over a long time/distance	
• Marathon running [3, 4]	• Lower extremity (tibialis anterior, plantar fascia, achilles) strains and tendinitis and ankle injuries [5] and stress fractures [6] in running and endurance athletes • Muscle fatigue of invertors or dorsiflexors can have a significant effect on the loading rates, peak magnitudes and ankle joint motion during running [7]
• Sailing [8]	• High repetition activities of hiking, pumping, grinding and steering are the major causes of overuse injury in experienced sailors who are fatigued [9]
• Rowing [10]	• Repetitive actions of the upper-body lead to lumbar and thoracic injuries such as joint and ligament sprains and tendinopathies [11]
Sports of shorter duration but with particularly repetitive sustained movements	
• Cricket •	• Fast bowlers, in particular, have been shown to be at high risk of back injuries due to repetitive lumbar hyperextension [12-16]
• Baseball and softball	• Pitchers delivering large numbers of balls to baseballers/softballers sustain serious overuse injuries be related to high physical workload and associated fatigue [17] • Rotator cuff injuries arise because the internal rotators experience high performance demand during pitching [17, 18]
• Dancers	• Repetitive movements, and high physical loads, experienced by dancers leads to joint and ligament injuries related to fatigue [19]
• Gymnasts	• Have repetitive movements, and high physical loads, that lead to joint and ligament injuries related to fatigue [20]
Sports with intense competition over a short bout	
• Football codes (soccer, rugby league, rugby union, Australian football, Gaelic football, etc)	• The injuries most commonly reported to be related to fatigue are to the lower limb and are muscle injuries or joint/ligament tears [21-29]
• Ice hockey	• Higher injury rates at the end of a tournament when player reaction times are slower due to fatigue [30]
Sports with a long playing season, such as many team sports	
• Football codes over 20+ week seasons	• Studies of various football codes in which injury rates have been shown to be different at different time points in the season [31-33]

Table 2 summarizes the broad approaches to how fatigue was measured or assessed in the epidemiological studies. As shown, of the studies that did include some measure of fatigue, none included a physiological measure of fatigue. Some examples of studies under each major category of fatigue measurement are expanded upon below for illustrative purposes. The major limitations of the types of study are also summarised in Table 2.

Table 2. Measurement of fatigue in epidemiological sports injury studies

Type of fatigue measure		
Features	**Study examples**	**Limitations of these measures and studies based on them**
Objective physiological or cognitive measures		
	• None	• No study reported use of these measures
No measures reported		
Mention of fatigue does not feature in methods or results sections of paper	• Most studies	• Opinion only, not evidence-based • Fatigue is just mentioned as a possible explanation for the findings in the discussion
Subjective measures only		
Self-report questionnaire based on psychological measures	• Profile of Mood States [35, 39] • Brunel Mood Scale [34]	• In studies which have applied a questionnaire measure after injury, it is not possible to tell if the fatigue scores are just the result of the current injury rather than the cause of injury • Studies which have only measured fatigue states at baseline may not show a fatigue effect because this would not manifest itself until later in a playing season
Proxy measures only		
High workload (particularly training)	• [3, 8, 10, 15, 20, 23, 36-38, 40]	• The player workload, particularly the time spent in training sessions has been recorded • Conclusions are drawn that athletes with higher training loads are more at risk of injury than others and therefore this is most likely due to fatigue resulting from excessive training loads
Short rest periods	• [15, 36, 41, 42]	• The number of rest days (or weeks) that athletes have had has been used to infer that players with a larger number of days of rest are less fatigued than those without so much rest
Time-of-season	• [19, 32, 33, 43-47]	• Injury incidence is described according to the time in the season when they occurred • Vast majority of these studies have been conducted in team sports, particularly the football codes • Association links made between higher injury rates at the end of a season and fatigue • No consistent time-of-season effects over a season in the same sports • Suggestions that higher injury rates at the start of the season could reflect lower levels of fitness in players at this stage, that would make them more susceptible to fatigue effects and hence injury • All conclusions drawn about injury risk and fatigue are from observational associations patterns linking time-of-season effects and it is not possible to link them temporally in time order to determine cause and effect relationships • Most important limitation is the fact that time-of-season effects, particularly at the end of season, can be explained by many other factors, other than fatigue; - differences in the intensity of the competition - players playing with recurrent or unrecovered previous injury

Type of fatigue measure		
Features	**Study examples**	**Limitations of these measures and studies based on them**
		- motivational factors such as a strong desire to win and push performance limits, to play with injury to make sure one is in a finals' team or, if playing in a team that will not make the finals, to play more recklessly or less carefully - a combination of the above
Phase-of-play		
	[4, 28-30, 32, 33, 43-46, 48-50]	• It is in inferred that differences across play phases (e.g. first quarter versus final quarter of a game) are indicative of fatigue levels in players, largely because the longer players play for the more tired they are likely to be • Reported in both team sports (e.g. football games) and in sporting events that occur over a large period of time, such as a marathon, with an increased number of conditions requiring medical attention as the competition distance increases • Major limitation is that there are also many other possible explanations for a higher injury rate at different stages of a game other than fatigue: - players with pre-existing, recurrent or unrecovered previous injury - accumulation of musculoskeletal microtrauma during a game - intensity of a game towards the end of a match (especially when the competition outcome is close) - players' reduced skill and decision making abilities in the latter parts of a game - motivational factors e.g. a strong desire to win and push performance limits, to play with injury to make sure one is in a finals' team or, if playing in a team that will not win, to play more recklessly or less carefully; or a combination of these.

Epidemiological Studies Relating Fatigue to Injury Incidence

Most of the 61 identified studies involved prospective surveillance of injuries over a playing season, with a small number reporting injuries over a few years. The majority of studies (about 70%) reported injury data that had been collected prospectively by trained data collectors (often physicians, physiotherapists, athletic trainers, etc). The remaining studies used a retrospective recall method through asking players/athletes to self-report their injuries. In these latter studies, the quality of the injury data is seriously hindered.

Almost all studies failed to consider the nature of the causal pathway between fatigue and injury and whether fatigue is a specific risk factor or injury risk effect modifier. Many studies grouped different types of injuries which increases the numbers of injuries in a study, but may bias the findings towards the null through a dilution of specific risk factor effects for different types of injury. Most studies have combined acute/traumatic and chronic/overuse factors even though their mechanisms and causal relationships with fatigue are likely to be different. A small number of studies considered specific types of injury, e.g. anterior cruciate ligament (ACL) injuries.

Measurement of Fatigue

Subjective ratings are the only current direct measure of fatigue; however, their subjective nature makes this measure vulnerable to various forms of bias. In studies outside the area of sport, fatigue is usually inferred from exposures known to cause it or at least make it more likely: factors relating to sleep (loss or poor quality), time of day and task are treated as causes of fatigue because they have been demonstrated to consistently make people feel tired. Ideally, studies should include both causal or 'proxy' measures and subjective measures.

Studies with No Fatigue Measures

The vast majority of studies (>85%) did not measure fatigue in any form but inferred its effects post hoc. For example, a study of injuries in America's Cup yacht racing over periods of varying training and sailing intensities showed injuries were most common during high training/moderate sailing followed by moderate training/high sailing periods [8]. The authors suggested a possible role of fatigue in injury causation due to long working days and little recovery time between activities. Unfortunately, the study included no measure of fatigue to substantiate this claim.

Studies with Psychological Measures of Fatigue

A study of 845 elite athletes across all sports used a self-report 374 item health screening questionnaire including the Brunel Mood Scale – fatigue subscale and retrospective recall of injuries over the previous 12 months [34]. Fatigue scores were significantly higher in currently-injured athletes compared to not-injured athletes, however the study was limited by a likely recall bias affecting coding of injuries and classification of injury status.

Another study conducted prospective injury surveillance, especially of ACL injuries, over 5 years in elite ballet and modern dancers [19]. All dancers completed the Profile of Mood States (POMS) at baseline and again at the time of injury reporting. While only a very small number of ACL injuries (n=12) were recorded, there were no differences in baseline POMS in ACL-injured and non-ACL injured dancers, but ACL-injured dancers had a significantly increased POMS fatigue score between baseline and time of injury. This study also recorded the time-of-day or season corresponding to the injury and found that nine of the 12 ACL injuries occurred towards the middle-end of performance season, leading the authors to suggest a possible link with fatigue. The POMS was also used in a study in varsity footballers and rugby players [35]. No significant relationship was found between the fatigue/inertia subscale and injury rates but fatigue was only measured at baseline or start of season so this is not surprising, since sport-related fatigue effects are more likely to occur as the playing season progresses.

Studies with Proxy Measures of Fatigue

Workload and Rest Breaks Effects

A number of studies have attributed effects of high workload and short rest breaks on injury to increased fatigue. When injury rates were compared over four consecutive professional British rugby league seasons, differences were explained by the overall season lengths and insufficient number of recovery days between games [36]. Similarly, when the playing season was increased from 21-23 games to about 29 games per season, higher rugby league injury incidence rates were reported [37]. Injury rates have also been reportedly higher at the start of a pre-season training period in soccer and attributed to the rapid increase in training workload [23].

A study of rugby union players [38] showed a relationship between injury severity during matches which was attributed to individual differences in capacity to withstand higher training volumes and to recover from any associated fatigue effects. Similarly, another study found that gymnasts from clubs that practiced for >20hrs/wk had significantly higher injury rates and cited fatigue was a major reason [20]. Further, a recent study of overuse injuries in 129 elite fast bowlers found that the impact of high workload was apparent three to four weeks later in increased injury rates [41]. Other studies have attributed links between workload related factors and injury to fatigue, including a review of marathon running injuries [3], America's Cup yacht racing [8], and rowing injuries [10].

The effect of rest was studied in junior cricket high performance fast bowlers [15]. The bowlers kept a daily diary of bowling workload (i.e. no. of match and training deliveries) and injuries (validated by a physiotherapist) over a playing session. Over the season, 25 percent of players reported an overuse injury although they were distributed equally across the playing season suggesting there was no time-of-season effect. However, the injured bowlers had bowled significantly more frequently than uninjured bowlers, with only 3.2 days rest on average since the last bowling episode compared to an average of 3.9 days for uninjured bowlers. This led the authors to conclude that the injured bowlers were not fully rested due to the reduced rest period and likely to still be in a fatigued state when they resumed their bowling.

Further evidence for a role of fatigue in injury risk comes from studies of changes in training loads. A rugby league study [40] showed that reductions in training loads reduced the rate of training injuries, whilst at the same time improving fitness levels in players. Another rugby league study suggested that an increased injury rate could have been influenced by a reduced pre-season break [42].

Time-of-season Effects

Because of a postulated effect of high workload on injury rates over several weeks, one study in cricket fast bowlers concluded that when monitoring overuse injuries, it may be more important to monitor season effects rather than just time-of-session [41]. In another study, match and training injuries reported in 156 semi-professional rugby league players over two consecutive seasons [32] tended to be more common towards the end of the season and training injuries more common towards the start of the season, with fatigue put forward as an explanation for both findings. Gabbett [24] reviewed injury incidence in rugby league players and concluded that in senior amateur and semi-professionals, match injuries occurred most commonly in the latter half of the season [32, 33], but conflicting evidence was found for time-of-season effects for professional players [25].

A study based on 6-month injury recall by elite Gaelic footballers [31] reported 28% of players sustained injuries in the last month of the season (June) compared to the next highest frequency of 19% in April. The authors explained these results in terms of ground condition changes over the season and the intensity of the competition towards the end of the season, though neither was measured objectively. Clearly, there is no single easy explanation for the time-of-season effect. In fact, the same evidence can be used to explain the relationship between ground hardness and injury risk and fatigue and injury risk [47, 51]. When there is an early-season bias in injury rates, authors have been more likely to suggest that ground conditions could explain this [52]. Direct measures of fatigue are needed to separate these explanations.

Phase-of-play Effects

Phase-of-play has also been linked to fatigue effects. Prospective injury surveillance was conducted in seven Finnish hockey teams for all games over two consecutive seasons [30]. The number of injuries was significantly higher in the third (or last) period of the game and the authors suggested that this was most likely to be related to changes in the intensity of the game and slower player reaction times associated with game fatigue. In a review of rugby-league injuries [24], the phase-of-play effect differed according to the level of play; in senior amateurs, more than 70% of the injuries occurred in the second half of the match [33], compared to 39% in semi-professionals [32] while injury rates were similar in both halves for professional players [25]. In one of the few studies to consider contact and non-contact injuries separately, a higher rate of contact match injuries occurred in the second half of a European Championship game which was attributed to reduced player focus associated with fatigue towards the end of a game [29]. As with the time-of-season studies, all of these conclusions are based solely on associations between injury incidence rates and time in game, without any actual assessment of fatigue across those phases.

A Model for How Fatigue and Injury Risk Could be Related

A number of authors have proposed multifactorial models for sports injury prevention [53,54] largely drawn from a mechanistic perspective of sports injury aetiology. A model of the psychological factors that impact on sports injuries included fatigue as one component of emotional state, but did not consider either physical fatigue or other mechanistic risk factors leading to sports injury [55]. Drawing on the Bahr and Holme [53] model, Figure 1 indicates the potential points where fatigue could possibly mediate injury risk and impact on the chain of events leading to sports injury.

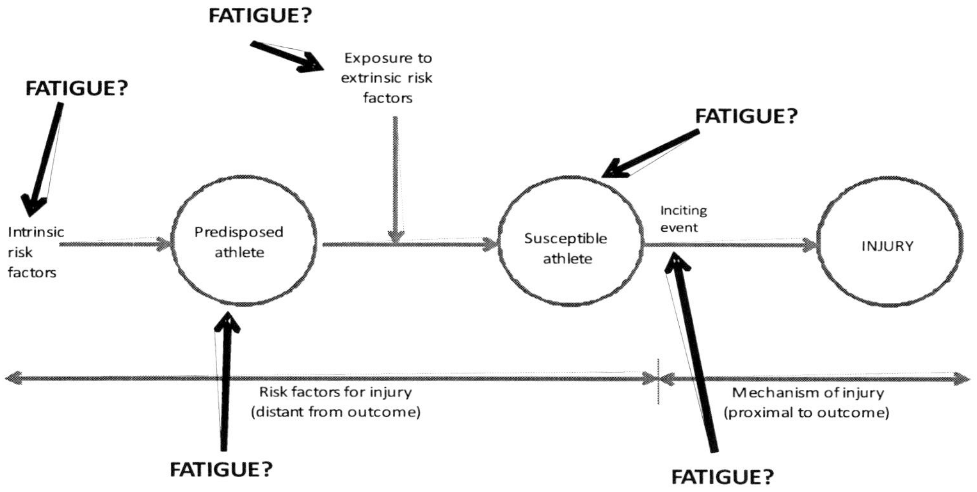

Figure 1. Potential points of action for fatigue effects to impact on aspects of the Bahr and Holme [53] aetiological model for injury causation.

Evidence for a Link between Fatigue, Decreased Sports Performance and Increased Injury Risk

The above review suggests a limited epidemiological evidence-base for the link between fatigue and injury during sport and exercise. Most of it is speculative, as no study combined direct measures of fatigue and investigation of factors thought to increase it. The vast majority of conclusions are based on statistical associations only. Given this, other sources of evidence linking fatigue to injury risk need to be considered. This section broadens the discussion about the putative for relationship between fatigue and injury by summarizing the evidence for the effects of fatigue on injury risk through decreased sports performance.

There is considerable literature on the relationship between fatigue and injury in a wide range of settings outside the field of sport (see [1] for a review). The general nature of the relationship is conceptualised as involving one or more factors known to cause the characteristic effects of fatigue including subjective feelings of tiredness and disinclination to continue, lowered muscle activity, decreased alertness and increased sleepiness. The fatigue induced by these causal factors in turn decreases the capacity to perform and it is these changes in performance that increase the likelihood of injury. This general model is depicted in Figure 2.

Physiological and Biomechanical Evidence Linking Fatigue and Injury

Based largely on laboratory-based investigations, a number of studies have suggested mechanisms that could link fatigue to the occurrence of musculoskeletal injuries during sport. These include decreases in muscle strength [56, 57]; muscle fatigue itself and its impact on reaction time [58], impaired joint position sense [59, 60]; delayed neuromuscular responses [59]; altered motor control strategies that then increase forces and strains on joints [61]; substantial degradation in both peripheral and central processing mechanisms [62]; reduced decision making where poor perceptions, decisions, reactions and resultant movement strategies may be more likely [62]; altered movement biomechanics that then impact on muscle flexibility, muscular strength, and body mechanics [63]; changes in ground reaction forces associated with altered running cadence, step length, and lower-extremity joint kinematics [64]; and negative effects on dynamic stability [65].

Intense or prolonged skeletal muscle contraction in sports inevitably results in a decline in muscle performance. It has been hypothesised that the physiological mechanisms associated with the decline in muscle performance in a fatigued state can also predispose athletes to injury. Unfortunately, this remains largely a hypothesis because of the difficulty in conducting appropriate studies, due to the obvious ethical issue of inducing harm in people. The size of the knowledge gap is further compounded as the physiological mechanisms of fatigue are clearly task-specific and multi-factorial in nature [66]. Nonetheless, data from several studies provide invaluable insight into likely causes of injury from exercise-induced fatigue.

Fatigued muscle has a reduced capability to absorb energy. Rabbit extensor digitorum muscle fatigued to 50% of its original maximal torque was compared to the contra-lateral muscle (non-fatigued) on the ability to resist stretch before tearing [67]. Whilst both muscles tore at the same length when stretched at three different rates, the fatigued muscle tear was able to absorb only 69-93% of the force of the contra-lateral muscle. In a second investigation [67], rabbit muscle tension was increased from none to 50% peak, and in other muscle, tension was decreased from 100% to 50% peak tension before being stretched to failure. Despite the different fatigue stimulus, the muscle tension, length and energy absorbed to failure was similar, indicating the contractile apparatus and properties play a role in muscle failure irrespective of fatigue mechanism.

Another likely physiological change linking fatigue to injury is motor control loss. People's ability to maintain balance on an unstable platform in synchrony with a visual tracking task was measured before and after fatigue-inducing isokinetic stair stepping exercise [68]. The ability to balance was significantly reduced after exercise indicating that motor control was impaired in the fatigued state. Several researchers argue that a reduction in motor control will increase the risk of ACL rupture, particularly in the landing phase of jumping, as a consequence of inadequate joint stabilisation and sub-optimal muscle activation strategy [68, 69].

The cause of the loss of motor control can reside "peripherally" or "centrally". In vitro, a decrease in pH reduces muscle spindle regulation of muscle stretch, resulting in greater muscle tremor [70]. Recent research suggests that motor loss could also be "central". In one experiment [69], unilateral single leg jumps to fatigue resulted in more extended hip & knee landing posture and increased landing loads in exercised and the contra-lateral leg (non-fatigued leg). These data suggest a "cross-over effect" of fatigue from the exercised to non-exercised leg that must be mediated within the central nervous system.

Hamstring tears constitute a significant problem for ball-sport athletes, accounting for 12-16% of total injuries in soccer (cited in [71]). The mechanistic causes of hamstring injury have received considerable attention, with specific focus on the ability to maintain eccentric strength in a fatigued state [57, 71, 72]. It is hypothesised that a fatigued-induced decrease in hamstring peak eccentric torque can increase injury susceptibility. Furthermore, it is suggested that a shift in peak eccentric torque to a shorter length may also compound injury risk. Therefore in a lengthened state that occurs in the deceleration phase of the swing phase of the running cycle the hamstrings may be less able to absorb force and therefore prone to tearing [71]. Whilst the precise cause of hamstring tears is elusive, the evidence supporting the fatigue theory is growing. Indeed after 90 minutes of performing a soccer-specific running task, hamstring eccentric peak torque decreases more and at a shorter length than quadriceps peak torque. Furthermore, these changes are more pronounced after "half-time" and coincide with a greater injury frequency in the latter states of play [72].

Whilst the precise mechanisms for physical fatigue-related increases in injury susceptibility are currently elusive, evidence is sufficient to experiment with specific injury-prevention interventions, especially strategies to sustain balance, limb biomechanics and hamstring peak torque.

Cognitive Effects of Fatigue and Injury Risk

Three groups of causal factors for cognitive or central fatigue have been identified: sleep deprivation, time-of-day and the nature of activity being undertaken. This section summarises the evidence for the fatigue effects of each of these causal factors on sports performance with subsequent inferred increased injury risk.

Time-of-day Effects

The effects of time-of-day on the body clock, physiological functions and performance are well-recognised [73, 74]. Most functions show a peak in the late afternoon to early evening and a trough in the early morning hours between 0200hrs and 0600hrs although there is some debate about the peak for injury [75]. The time-of-day effects relevant to sport are mainly through the timing of competition and the effects of time-shifts/jetlag due to competition in different time zones.

There are a number of reviews of time-of-day or circadian effects on exercise or sports performance. Increasing need for sports to be played at times when the body is usually asleep, such as tennis tournaments that extend into the early hours of the morning, make the consideration of time-of-day effects increasingly important. Most, but not all, attributes of sports performance vary with time-of-day, mirroring the circadian rhythm and peaking in the early evening [76]. Moreover, time-of-day effects probably occur for strength, anaerobic power and capacity, body temperature and exercise response, but are less clear for endurance training, ratings of perceived exertion, arm exercise and self-paced exercise [77]. For example, performance was found to vary with time-of-day in soccer players tested at 0800, 1200, 1600 and 2000hrs [78]. Self-rated alertness and fatigue were highest at 2000hrs but not all performance measures showed time-of-day changes and the peak for different performance measures varied.

Time-of-day effects on swim performance were found to peak between 5-7 hours before the circadian rhythm nadir (around 2300hrs) and were poorest one hour either side of the nadir (around 0500hrs) indicating a circadian rhythm in laboratory-based sports performance independent of sleep or environmental factors [79]. A comprehensive review of the evidence argued that there is sufficient evidence that time-of-day has an effect on athletes' performance, but the specific nature of these effects are not clear, especially what aspects of performance are affected, or whether particular types of sports are more vulnerable [80].

One of the only sports injury-specific studies to examine time-of-day effects is a recent study in dancers [19]. Although based on only a small number of ACL (n=12) injuries, the authors reported that three-quarters of these injuries occurred in the evening and concluded that the higher evening rate was a consequence of sustained activity during the day. This finding could also be explained by the fact that, in the evenings, dancers gave professional performances and so may have been at injury risk for other reasons.

Jetlag due to transmeridian travel is a specific type of disruption to the circadian rhythm and most likely to produce time-of-day effects on performance [81]. One review concluded that jetlag produced symptoms relevant to sports performance like fatigue and difficulties with concentrating, but presented no evidence for performance effects [82]. Other studies concluded that more research is needed to identify the effects of transmeridian travel on performance [76] or argued that the evidence for jetlag effects is inconclusive because the quality of the studies are too poor [80].

A significant problem with studies of time-of-day effects is that they are often the result of both time-of-day and sleep deprivation; the tennis player playing the fourth set of an important tournament at 0100hrs has been awake for long hours so making it difficult to draw conclusions about the independent effects of these factors. The issue especially applies to jetlag effects where athletes are tired due to a long journey as well as in a different time zone.

Sleep Deprivation Effects

Sleep deprivation is one of the most obvious reasons for experiencing fatigue. There is good evidence from many studies that reduced quantity or quality of sleep or more time awake produces sleep debt and a homeostatic need for sleep [83]. This produces decrements in alertness and performance and increases the likelihood of injury (see Figure 2). In sport, these effects can occur where external influences disrupt sleep such as sleeping in unfamiliar quarters or due to jetlag or where shortened sleep occurs due to early morning starts or late bedtimes due to competing demands of exercise, work, social and family life.

A recent review of the effects of sleep loss concluded that the behavioural and biological effects of sleep loss are well-recognised in many settings and this should also apply to sport [78]. The authors argue that the consequences of sleep-loss related errors in performance could be as important for sports activities involving physical contact as for aviation or in industrial settings.

A few studies have examined the effects of acute sleep loss on exercise performance. Weightlifting performance was compared after 24 hours without sleep and one night of normal sleep [84]; the former had increased self-ratings of fatigue but no performance effects. The authors concluded that acute sleep deprivation could have adverse effects on performance due to psychological or motivational influences.

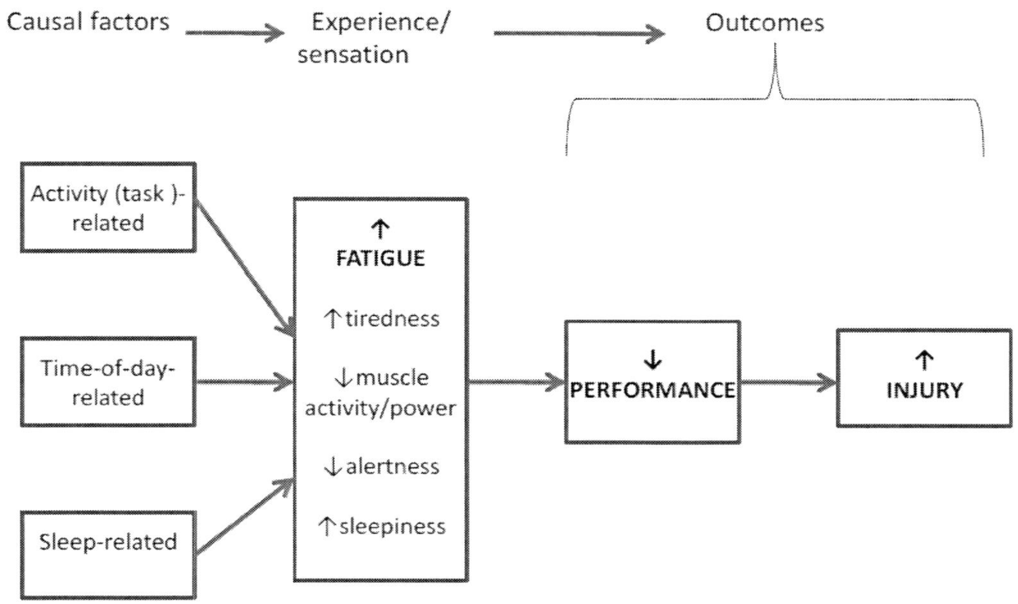

Figure 2. The theoretical relationship between the primary causes of fatigue, the experience of fatigue and performance and injury outcomes.

Other studies of total sleep deprivation showed no or only moderate effects on exercise performance. Over 42 hours of sleep deprivation, naval seaman reported feeling fatigued but showed only small decrements in naval tasks requiring gross motor activity [85]. Exercise performance decrements were found over a longer period without sleep where players in an endurance soccer match lasting nearly 92 hours showed significant reductions in activity and exercise heart rate [86]. In contrast, a laboratory study comparing runners and volleyball players over a period of 25-30 hours without sleep to rested controls showed that sleep loss reduced: exercise minute ventilation, resting carbon dioxide production in both groups, time to exercise exhaustion in volleyballers, and resting oxygen uptake in runners [87]. Another study found that the amount of habitual exercise had little effect on individual differences in subjective and physical performance after one night without sleep, with effects only for subjective mood states [88].

There is some evidence of the effects of partial sleep loss on exercise performance. Studies of endurance exercise such as solo Atlantic crossings (84) and adventure racing (85) showed significant increases in state anxiety and fatigue with increasing sleep deprivation. Laboratory studies of the effects of reduced sleep on dart throwing and weight lifting also increasing fatigue ratings and performance decrements [89]. The importance of adequate sleep can also be inferred from studies of napping. A study of the effects of a post-lunch nap after a night of shortened sleep [90] showed higher alertness and better sprint times indicating the importance of sleep for performance. The relationship between sleep loss and exercise may not be entirely straightforward. There is evidence of a reciprocal effect between sleep and exercise. While decreased sleep can produce decreased exercise performance on at least some dimensions, there is also evidence that physical activity and exercise can overcome the effects of sleep deprivation, at least over short periods. For example, during 30 hours of sleep deprivation reaction times were significantly faster where participants engaged in intermittent physical exercise than if they had simply rested [91].

Task-related Effects

The third major cause of fatigue comprises a range of task-related factors including the duration, intensity and frequency of exercise. Again, these factors are argued to cause fatigue with subsequent effects on performance and injury risk. A number of studies (e.g. [34, 92]) showed that psychological state, including fatigue, predicted athlete injury although often the assessment of fatigue was retrospective, so weakening the argument of a predictive relationship.

There is considerable laboratory research on the effect of fatigue caused by a single episode of high-intensity exercise on subsequent exercise performance. Much of this research focused on the effects of fatigue on specific functions of the lower limb, especially the knee. For example, pre/post exercise comparisons showed decreased maximal knee extension position and decreased stride rate [93], decreases in knee flexor strength [94, 95] and force [96] and reduced pre-activation of hamstrings and gastrocnemius muscles [97]. Similarly, exercise-induced fatigue has been shown to decrease motor control capacity as shown by measures of balance [68] which persisted for up to ten minutes [98]. A conclusion common to many of these studies was that the performance decrements signal increased injury risk.

There is some evidence that performance can be modified when fatigued, to mitigate the effects of high-intensity or long duration exercise which might increase injury risk. Changes like decreased knee flexion after an exhaustive running exercise [95] and impairment in voluntary peak flexion and faster neuromuscular response of the knee joint after maximal static exercise [96] have been interpreted as an effort to protect the knee from injury. Similarly the finding that compared to non-athletes, athletes were able to regulate inter-limb joint stiffness in a single-legged hopping protocol following fatigue-inducing repeated sprints [99] was attributed to training and would reduce athletes' injury risk. Clearly, more research is needed to determine whether the fatigue-related changes in neuromuscular function can reduce injury risk and whether training can enhance this effect.

Many of these studies do not take into account the way fatigue is induced. Many studies used a cardiovascular task or specific exercise protocol which would have produced both local muscular fatigue and general body fatigue (e.g. 63,92,98,99) whereas others induced only localised fatigue using non-cardiovascular exercise [96, 100]. The latter produces much lower effects of local fatigue and is unlikely to have effects on general or central fatigue. These studies therefore may not reflect real-world exercise conditions and the likelihood of injury.

It is also important to distinguish the fatiguing effects of exercise involving only a local anatomical area and fatigue with a more general effect due to the differences in the motivational and effort-related influences. One of the important characteristics of general or central fatigue is a disinclination to continue or to exert more effort [101] which is much less likely to occur when fatigue is localised to a particular muscle region where the muscle can be tired, but the incentive to continue to exert effort remains high. Declining effort will have enormous impact on exercise performance and can also reduce any attempts to protect against injury due to local fatigue effects. Studies of the effect of fatigue on performance and injury risk must attempt to control for these influences or at the least to measure their effects. The role of motivation and effort must be included in studies of the effects of fatigue on exercise performance.

CONCLUSION

While the above text has treated physiological fatigue and each of the three major causes of cognitive fatigue as independent factors, in the real-world context of sports performance these factors rarely occur in isolation. High performance athletes faced with long duration or high intensity blocks of exercise are often also fatigued because they could not sleep the previous night or because they had to cross a number of time zones to participate in the competition. It is almost certain that sleep and time-of-day effects on fatigue are accumulative. The question of how these factors interact with task-related factors has hardly been asked. There is clearly much opportunity for further research on these questions.

Table 3. Research priorities and directions for future epidemiological studies linking fatigue and its sports performance deficits to injury risk

Research Theme/topic	
Questions that need answering	**Sub-questions/comparisons/ approaches**
Injury types	
• Is it meaningful to combine all injury types in one study? (e.g. end of season effects disappear when only looking at hamstring injuries [102] • Is the role of fatigue likely to be the same for all injury mechanisms?	• different body regions/tissues may respond to fatigue inputs and effects differently • acute/traumatic versus chronic/overuse
Measurement of fatigue	
• Could an injury criterion be developed that rates the likelihood of injury risk to fatigue? • How could measures of fatigue be incorporated? • How good are the proxy measures of fatigue in prospective epidemiological studies and could they be improved? • How good are subjective measures of fatigue in prospective epidemiological sports injury studies and could they be improved?	• e.g. very likely to be related to fatigue; possibly related to fatigue; unlikely to be related to fatigue; unknown • as baseline measures • as factors measured over time • without confounding of the cause/effect of injury
Risk factors	
• Do time-of-season and phase-of-play effects really reflect fatigue? • At what point/s in the injury chain is fatigue likely to operate? Does this differ by type of injury or injury mechanism? • How can the independent effect of fatigue be assessed in relation to other possible risk factors?	• time of season • phase of play • workload effects, including delayed effects • accumulated workload, overload

Table 3. (Continued)

Analysis of fatigue measures	
• What is the relationship between objective, subjective and proxy measures of fatigue?	• all studies have looked at proxy or other measures of fatigue uni-variably (i.e. without adjustment for other factors)
• How does fatigue relate to, or act in combination with, the other possible factors leading to injury?	• independent effect (adjusting for other factors) • covariate (one of many factors) • effect modifier (factor modifying effect of others)
• How, and which, novel statistical approaches towards analysing sports injury data be used?	• structural equation modelling • including time-variant covariates in regression models as baseline measures • generalised estimating equations, accounting for structural clustering

Overall, there is good evidence that lack of sleep for a variety of reasons can have adverse effects on exercise performance, which are likely to increase injury risk. Further research is needed to explore the critical characteristics of sleep loss that are important and the nature of the performance decrement and links with injury for particular types of exercise. In general, task-related factors can clearly influence exercise performance in a number of complex ways. It is not clear, however, whether these changes reflect adverse effects on performance or are attempts to counteract the effects of fatigue on performance which are precursors to injury or increase injury risk. It is also not clear whether a bout of exercise could be used to overcome the effects of fatigue. We need the answers to these questions, but studies with much better designs are needed to clarify how task-related fatigue, exercise performance and injury risk are related. As stated by Brooks et al. [43], even though the pattern of injuries according to phase (or time)-of-play might suggest fatigue as a possible contributing factor "it is difficult to identify specific central or peripheral causes". Until epidemiological studies formally measure both fatigue and these other factors over time and link them with high quality protective injury surveillance, any causal relationships with fatigue will be at best speculative.

This Chapter has shown that there is accumulating evidence from the experimental literature about the effect of fatigue on performance in sport, with implications of this for injury risk. There is also a large international literature about the role of fatigue and sleep deprivation in injury risk in broader injury contexts that could be used to inform further research in sports fatigue and injury risk studies. To date, no prospective epidemiological sports injury study published in the peer-reviewed literature has explored the potential link between fatigue and sports injury risk properly. When fatigue has been identified as a factor in sports injury risk, it is generally solely in terms of an association between observed injury incidence patterns and the phase-of-play or time-of-season when the injury occurred. Most importantly, whilst epidemiological studies may state or conclude that fatigue is a likely or possible injury risk factor, no study has yet adequately measured fatigue and directly related these measures to injury incidence.

Overall, this Chapter highlights a need to conduct further epidemiological research in this area, especially as there is evidence for underlying cognitive and physiological mechanisms of fatigue having an impact of injury outcomes in athletes. Specific suggestions for a future research agenda, adopting a truly multidisciplinary research strategy in epidemiologically-focussed studies, are outlined in Table 3.

Taken together, the evidence presented in this Chapter suggests that fatigue does increase injury risk in sport. However, we need many more studies using optimal study designs such as prospective cohort studies to be sure. These studies will also be necessary to more confidently define when and why fatigue-related sports injuries occur.

ACKNOWLEDGMENTS

Caroline Finch was supported by a National Health and Medical Research Council (NHMRC) Principal Research Fellowship and Ann Williamson was supported by an NHMRC Senior Research Fellowship. The authors would like to thank Lucy Millar for providing research assistance support in identifying studies for including in this review. The Australian Centre for Research into Injury in Sport and its Prevention (ACRISP) is one of the International Research Centres for Prevention of Injury and Protection of Athlete Health supported by the Internatonal Olympic Committee (IOC).

REFERENCES

[1] Williamson A, Lombardi DA, Folkard S, Stutts J, Courtney TK, Connor JL. The link between fatigue and safety. *Accid Anal Prev*, 2011, 43, 498-515.

[2] Cochrane Injuries Group. Systematic reviews of interventions for preventing sleep-related injuries. *Injury Prev*, 2009, 15, 428.

[3] Fredericson M, Misra A. Epidemiology and aetiology of marathon running injuries. *Sports Med*, 2007, 37, 437-9.

[4] Dallam G, Jonas S, Miller T. Medical considerations in triathlon competition: recommendations for triathlon organisers, competitors and coaches. *Sports Med*, 2005, 35, 143-61.

[5] Reber L, Perry J, Pink M. Muscular control of the ankle in running. *Am J Sports Med*, 1993, 21, 805-10.

[6] Weist R, Eils E, Rosenbaum D. The influence of muscle fatigue on electromyogram and plantar pressure patterns as an explanation for the incidence of metatarsal stress fractures. *Am J Sports Med*, 2004, 32, 1893-8.

[7] Christina KA, White SC, Gilchrist LA. Effect of localized muscle fatigue on vertical ground reaction forces and ankle joint motion during running. *Hum Mov Sci*, 2001, 20, 257-76.

[8] Neville V, Molloy J, JHM B, Speedy D, Atkinson G. Epidemiology of injuries and illness in America's Cup yacht racing. *Br J Sports Med*, 2006, 40, 304-12.

[9] Neville V, Folland J. The epidemiology and aetiology of injuries in sailing. *Sports Med*, 2009, 39, 129-45.

[10] Rumball J, Lebrun C, DiCiacca S, Orlando K. Rowing injuries. *Sports Med*, 2006, 35, 537-55.

[11] Hickey G, Fricker P, McDonald W. Injuries to elite rowers over a 10-yr period. *Med Sci Sports Exerc*, 1997, 20, 1567-72.
[12] Gerrard DF. Overuse injury and growing bones: the young athlete at risk. *Br J Sports Med*, 1993, 27, 14-8.
[13] Foster D, Elliott B, Ackland T, Fitch K. Back injuries to fast bowlers in cricket: a prospective study. *Br J Sports Med*, 1989, 23, 150-4.
[14] Dennis R, Farhart P, Clements M, Ledwidge H. The relationship between fast bowling workload and injury in first-class cricketers: a pilot study. *J Sci Med Sport*, 2004, 7, 232-6.
[15] Dennis R, Finch C, Farhart P. Is bowling workload a risk factor for injury to Australian junior cricket fast bowlers? *Br J Sports Med*, 2005, 39, 843-6.
[16] Dennis R, Finch C, McIntosh A, Elliott B. Using field-based tests to identify injury risk factors for fast bowlers in cricket. *Br J Sports Med*, 2008, 42, 477-82.
[17] Flyger N, Button C, Rishraj N. The science of softball: implications for performance and injury prevention. *Sports Med*, 2006, 36, 797-816.
[18] Mullaney M, McHugh P, Donofrio T, Nicholas S. Upper and lower extremity muscle fatigue after a baseball pitching performance. *Am J Sports Med*, 2005, 33, 108-13.
[19] Liederbach M, Dilgen F, Rose D. Incidence of anterior cruciate ligament injuries among elite ballet and modern dancers. *Am J Sports Med*, 2008, 36, 1779-88.
[20] Pettrone F, Ricciardelli E. Gymnastic injuries: the Virginia experience 1982-1983. *Am J Sports Med*, 1987, 15, 59-62.
[21] Keller C, Noyes F, Buncher C. The medical aspects of soccer injury epidemiology. *Am J Sports Med*, 1987, 15, 230-7.
[22] Chomiak J, Junge A, Peterson L, Dvorak J. Severe injuries in football players. Influencing factors. *Am J Sports Med*, 2000, 28, S58-S68.
[23] Woods C, Hawkins R, Hulse M, Hodson A. The Football Association Medical Research Programme: an audit of injuries in professional football-analysis of preseason injuries. *Br J Sports Med*, 2002, 36, 436-41.
[24] Gabbett TJ. Incidence of injury in junior and senior rugby league players. *Sports Med*, 2004, 34, 849-59.
[25] Gabbett TJ. Influence of training and match intensity on injuries in rugby league. *J Sports Sci*, 2004, 22, 409-17.
[26] Gabbett T, Domrow N. Relationships between training load, injury, and fitness in sub-elite collision sport athletes. *J Sports Sci*, 2007, 25, 1507-19.
[27] Gabbe B, Finch C, Wajswlener H, Bennell K. Predictors of hamstring injuries at the elite-level of Australian football. *Scand J Sci Med Sport*, 2006, 16, 7-13.
[28] Best J, McIntosh A, Savage T. Rugby World Cup 2003 injury surveillance project. *Br J Sports Med*, 2005, 39, 812-7.
[29] Hagglund M, Walden M, Ekstrand J. UEFA injury study an injury audit of European Championships 2006 to 2008. *Br J Sports Med*, 2009, 43, 483-9.
[30] Molsa J, Airaksinen O, Nasman O, Torstila I. Ice hockey injuries in Finland: a prospective epidemiological study. *Am J Sports Med*, 1997, 24, 495-9.
[31] Cromwell F, Walsh J, Gormley J. A pilot study examining injuries in elite gaelic footballers. *Br J Sports Med*, 2000, 34, 104-8.
[32] Gabbett TJ. Incidence of injury in semi-professional rugby league players. *Br J Sports Med*, 2003, 37, 36-44.

[33] Gabbett TJ. Incidence, site, and nature of injuries in amateur rugby league over three consecutive seasons. *Br J Sports Med*, 2000, 34, 98-103.
[34] Galambos SA, Terry PC, Moyle GM, Locke SA. Psychological predictors of injury among elite athletes. *Br J Sports Med*, 2005, 39, 351-4.
[35] Lavallee L, Flint F. The relationship of stress, competitive anxiety, mood state, and social support to athletic injury. *J Athletic Train*, 1996, 31, 296-9.
[36] Hodgson-Phillips L, Standen P, Batt M. Effects of seasonal change in rugby league on the incidence of injury. *Br J Sports Med*, 1998, 32, 144-8.
[37] Gissane C, Jennings D, Kerr K, White J. Injury rates in rugby league football: Impact of change in playing season. *Am J Sports Med*, 2003, 31, 954-8.
[38] Brooks J, Fuller C, Kemp S, Reddin D. An assessment of training volume in professional rugby union and its impact on the incidence, severity, and nature of match and training injuries. *J Sports Sci*, 2008, 26, 863-73.
[39] Perna F, Antoni M, Baum A, Gordon P, Schneiderman N. Cognitive behavioural stress management effects on injury and illness among competitive athletes: a randomized clinical trial. *Ann Behav Med*, 2003, 25, 66-73.
[40] Gabbett T. Reductions in pre-season training loads reduce training injury rates in rugby league players. *Br J Sports Med*, 2004, 38, 743-9.
[41] Orchard J, James T, Kountouris A, Dennis R. Fast bowlers in cricket demonstrate up to 3- to 4- week delay between high workloads and increased risk of injury. *Am J Sports Med*, 2009, 37, 1186-92.
[42] Gissane C, Jennings D, White J, Cumine A. Injury in summer rugby league football: the experiences of one club. *Br J Sports Med*, 1998, 32, 149-52.
[43] Brook J, Fuller C, Kemp S, Reddin D. Epidemiology of injuries in English professional rugby union: part 1 match injuries. *Br J Sports Med*, 2005, 39, 757-66.
[44] Tscholl P, O'Riordan D, Fuller C, Dvorak J, Junge A. Tackle mechansims and match characteristics in women's elite football tournaments. *Br J Sports Med*, 2007, 41, i15-i9.
[45] Wilson F, Caffrey S, King E, Casey K, Gissane C. A 6-month prospective study of injury in Gaelic football. *Br J Sports Med*, 2007, 41, 317-21.
[46] Hawkins RD, Hulse MA, WIlkinson C, Hodson A, Gibson M. The association football medical research programme: an audit of injuries in professional football. *Br J Sports Med*, 2001, 35, 43-7.
[47] Walden M, Hagglund M, Ekstrand J. UEFA champions league study: a prospective study of injuries in professional football during the 2001-2002 season. *Br J Sports Med*, 2005, 39, 542-6.
[48] Yard E, Comstock R. Effects of field location, time in competition, and phase of play on injury severity in high school football. *Res Sports Med*, 2009, 17, 35-49.
[49] Dvorak J, Junge A, Grimm K, Kirkendall D. Medical report from the 2006 FIFA World Cup Germany. *Br J Sports Med*, 2007, 41, 578-81.
[50] Bottini E, Poggi EJT, Luzuriaga F, Secin FP. Incidence and nature of the most common rugby injuries sustained in Argentina (1991-1997). *Br J Sports Med*, 2000, 34, 94-7.
[51] Orchard J. Is there a relationship between ground and climatic conditions and injuries in football? *Sports Med*, 2002, 32, 419-32.
[52] Takemura M, Schneiders A, Bell M, Milburn P. The association of ground hardness with injuries in rugby union. *Br J Sports Med*, 2007, 41, 582-7.

[53] Bahr R, Holme I. Risk factors for sports injuries - a methodological approach. *Br J Sports Med*, 2003, 37, 384-92.

[54] Meeuwisse WH. Assessing causation in sport injury: a multifactorial model. *Clin J Sport Med*, 1994, 4, 166-70.

[55] Junge A. The influence of psychological factors on sports injuries: review of the literature. *Am J Sports Med*, 2000, 28, S10-S5.

[56] Nyland J, Shapiro R, Caborn D, Nitz A, Malone T. The effect of quadriceps femoris, hamstring, and placebo eccentric fatigue on knee and ankle dynamics during crossover cutting. *J Orthop Sports Phys Ther*, 1997, 25, 171-84.

[57] Rahnama N, Reilly T, Lees A, Graham-Smith P. Muscle fatigue induced by exercise simulating the work rate of competitive soccer. *J Sports Sci*, 2003, 21, 933-42.

[58] Davis J, Baliley S. Possible mechanisms of central nervous system fatigue during exercise. *Med Sci Sports Exerc*, 1997, 29, 45-57.

[59] Rozzi S, Lephart S, Gear W, Fu F. Knee joint laxity and neuromuscular characteristics of male and female soccer and basketball players. *Am J Sports Med*, 1999, 27, 312-9.

[60] Skinner HB, Wyatt MP, Hodgdon JA, Conard DW, Barrack RL. Effect of fatigue on joint position sense of the knee. *J Orth Res*, 1986, 4, 112-8.

[61] Chappell JD, Herman DC, Knight BS, Kirkendall DT, Garrett WE, Yu B. Effect of fatigue on knee kinetics and kinematics in stop-jump tasks. *Am J Sports Med*, 2005, 33, 1022-9.

[62] Borotikar BS, Newcomer R, Koppes R, McLean SG. Combined effects of fatigue and decision making on female lower limb landing postures: central and peripheral contributions to ACL injury risk. *Clin Biomech*, 2008, 23, 81-92.

[63] Small K, McNaughton LR, Greig M, Lohkamp M, Lovell R. Soccer fatigue, sprinting and hamstring injury risk. *Int J Sports Med*, 2009, 30, 573-8.

[64] Gerlach K, White S, Burton H, Dorn J, Leddy J, Horvath P. Kinetic changes with fatigue and relationship to injury in female runners. *Med Sci Sports Exerc*, 2005, 37, 657-63.

[65] Shaw M, Gribble P, Frye J. Ankle bracing, fatigue, and time to stabilization in collegiate volleyball athletes. *J Athletic Train*, 2008, 43, 164-71.

[66] Enoka RM, Duchateau J. Muscle fatigue: what, why and how it influences muscle function. *J Physiol*, 2008, 586, 11-23.

[67] Mair S, Seaber A, Glisson R, Garrett WJ. The role of fatigue in susceptibility to acute muscle strain injury. *Am J Sports Med*, 1996, 24, 137-43.

[68] Johnston RI, Howard M, Cawley P, Losse G. Effect of lower extremity muscular fatigue on motor control performance. *Med Sci Sports Exerc*, 1998, 30, 1703-7.

[69] McLean S, Samorezov J. Fatigue-induced ACL injury risk stems from a degradation in central control. *Med Sci Sports Exerc*, 2009, 41, 1661-72.

[70] Fischer M, Schafer S. Effects of changes in pH on the afferent impulse activity of isolated cat muscle spindles. *Brain Res*, 2005, 1043, 153-75.

[71] Small K, McNaughton L, Greig M, Lovell R. The effects of multidirectional soccer-specific fatigue on markers of hamstring injury risk. *J Sci Med Sport*, 2008, 13, 120-5.

[72] Greig M, Siegler J. Soccer-specific fatigue and eccentric hamstrings muscle strength. *J Athletic Train*, 2009, 44, 180-4.

[73] Czeisler CA, Weitzman ED, Moore-Ede MC, Zimmerman JC, Kronauer RS. Human sleep: its duration and organization depend on its circadian phase. *Sci*, 1980, 210, 1264-7.

[74] Zulley J, Wever RA, Aschoff J. The dependence of onset and duration of sleep on the circadian rhythm of rectal temperature. *Pflügers Arch*, 1981, 391, 314-8.

[75] Folkard S, Lombardi DA, Spencer MB. Estimating the circadian rhythm in the risk of occupational injuries and "accidents". *Chronobiol Int*, 2006, 23, 1181-92.

[76] Atkinson G, Reilly T. Circadian variation in sports performance. *Sports Med*, 1996, 21, 292-312.

[77] Cappaert TA. Time of day effect on athletic performance: An update. *J Strength Cond Res*, 1999, 13, 412-21.

[78] Reilly T, Edwards B. Altered sleep-wake cycles and physical performance in athletes. *Physiol Behav*, 2007, 90, 274-84.

[79] Kline CE, Durstine JL, Davis JM, Moore TA, Devlin TM, Zielinski MR, et al. Circadian variation in swim performance. *J Appl Physiol*, 2007, 102, 641-9.

[80] Reilly T, Waterhouse J. Sports performance: is there evidence that the body clock plays a role? *Eur J Appl Physiol*, 2009, 106, 321-32.

[81] Winget CM, DeRoshia CW, Holley DC. Circadian rhythms and athletic performance. *Med Sci Sports Exerc*, 1985, 17, 498-516.

[82] Manfredini R, Manfredini F, Fersini C, Conconi F. Circadian rhythms, athletic performance, and jet lag. *Br J Sports Med*, 1998, 32, 101-6.

[83] Van Dongen H, Maislin G. The cumulative cost of additional wakefulness: dose-response effects on neurobehavioral functions and sleep physiology from chronic sleep restriction and total sleep deprivation. *Sleep*, 2003, 26, 117-26.

[84] Blumert P, Crum A, Ernsting M, Volek J, Hollander D, Haff E, et al. The acute effects of twenty-four hours of sleep loss on the performance of national-caliber male collegiate weightlifters. *J Strength Cond Res*, 2007, 21, 1146-54.

[85] How JM, Foo SC, Low E, Wong TM, Vijayan A, Siew MG, et al. Effects of sleep deprivation on performance of Naval seamen: I. Total sleep deprivation on performance. *Ann Acad Med Singapore*, 1994, 23, 669-75.

[86] Reilly T, Walsh TJ. Physiological, psychological and performance measures during an endurance record for five-a-side soccer. *Br J Sports Med*, 1981, 15, 122-8.

[87] Azboy O, Kaygisiz Z. Effects of sleep deprivation on cardiorespiratory functions of the runners and volleyball players during rest and exercise. *Acta Physiol Hung*, 2009, 96, 29-36.

[88] Meney I, Waterhouse J, Atkinson G, Reilly T, Davenne D. The effect of one night's sleep deprivation on temperature, mood, and physical performance in subjects with different amounts of habitual physical activity. *Chronobiol Int*, 1998, 15, 349-63.

[89] Edwards BJ, Waterhouse J. Effects of one night of partial sleep deprivation upon diurnal rhythms of accuracy and consistency in throwing darts. *Chronobiol Int*, 2009, 26, 756-68.

[90] Waterhouse J, Atkinson G, Edwards B, Reilly T. The role of a short post-lunch nap in improving cognitive, motor, and sprint performance in participants with partial sleep deprivation. *J Sports Sci*, 2007, 25, 1557-66.

[91] Scott JP, McNaughton LR, Polman RC. Effects of sleep deprivation and exercise on cognitive, motor performance and mood. *Physiol Behav*, 2006, 87, 396-408.

[92] Devonport TJ, Lane AM, Hanin YL. Emotional states of athletes prior to performance-induced injury. *J Sports Sci Med*, 2005, 4, 382-94.

[93] Mizrahi J, Verbitsky O, Isakov E, Daily D. Effect of fatigue on leg kinematics and impact acceleration in long distance running. *Hum Mov Sci*, 2000, 19, 139-51.

[94] Greig M. The influence of soccer-specific fatigue on peak isokinetic torque production of the knee flexors and extensors. *Am J Sports Med*, 2008, 36, 1403-9.

[95] Benjaminse A, Habu A, Sell TC, Abt JP, Fu FH, Myers JB, et al. Fatigue alters lower extremity kinematics during a single-leg stop-jump task. *Knee Surg Sports Traumatol Arthrosc*, 2008, 16, 400-7.

[96] Minshull C, Gleeson N, Walters-Edwards M, Eston R, Rees D. Effects of acute fatigue on the volitional and magnetically-evoked electromechanical delay of the knee flexors in males and females. *Eur J Appl Physiol*, 2007, 100, 469-78.

[97] Gehring D, Melnyk M, Gollhofer A. Gender and fatigue have influence on knee joint control strategies during landing. *Clin Biomech*, 2009, 24, 82-7.

[98] Yaggie J, Armstrong WJ. Effects of lower extremity fatigue on indices of balance. *J Sport Rehab*, 2004, 13, 312-22.

[99] Clark RA. The effect of training status on inter-limb joint stiffness regulation during repeated maximal sprints. *J Sci Med Sport*, 2009, 12, 406-10.

[100] Apriantono T, Nunome H, Ikegami Y, Sano S. The effect of muscle fatigue on instep kicking kinetics and kinematics in association football. *J Sports Sci*, 2006, 24, 951-60.

[101] Hockey GRJ. Compensatory control in the regulation of human performance under stress and high workload: A cognitive-energetical framework. *Biol Psychol*, 1997, 45, 73-93.

[102] Gabbe B, Finch C, Bennell K, Wajswelner H. Risk factors for hamstring injuries in community-level Australian Football. *Br J Sports Med*, 2005, 39, 106-10.

In: Regulation of Fatigue in Exercise
Editor: Frank E. Marino
ISBN 978-1-61209-334-5

Chapter 10

FATIGUE – INSIGHTS FROM INDIVIDUAL AND TEAM SPORTS

David B. Pyne*, David T. Martin
Australian Institute of Sport, Department of Physiology, PO Box 176
Belconnen ACT 2616, Australia

ABSTRACT

Many different aspects of fatigue in sport have been researched, discussed and written about. However, the sport science practitioner can often find it difficult to access relevant and meaningful scientific evidence when it comes to managing training loads and fatigue effectively. Should training programs proceed as planned, be modified or cease altogether? These decisions are difficult and often left to the coach who may have many years of experience associated with managing fatigue in a productive way. This chapter addresses fatigue from a practical perspective and published research in this complex area. Fatigue in individual and team sports can present different challenges that have encouraged different approaches. There are certainly as many questions as answers when it comes to optimally managing a "fatigued" athlete. Continual research exploring the relationship between training patterns and performance ability is certainly warranted. The exciting area of recovery and fatigue dissipation is yielding many interesting and relevant findings. Fatigue induced by training – is most likely a pre-requisite for success in elite sport. However, the merits of excessive fatigue remain to be clarified. Practitioners working daily with elite athletes have the potential to guide important research for effective diagnosis and management of fatigue.

Email: david.pyne@ausport.gov.au

INTRODUCTION

Fatigue is an everyday issue for coaches, athletes and sports scientists in both individual and team sports. A colloquial expression holds that "training hard and managing fatigue on a daily basis is all part of being a highly trained athlete". Fatigue can be categorised as either short-term (acute) or long-term (chronic) depending on its duration and severity. A holistic model of fatigue is most commonly employed that accounts for both physiological and non-physiological factors in highly trained athletes. Technology and science evolve quickly but conditioning practices and philosophies in sport are often based on long-standing cultures and traditions. The historical approach for monitoring fatigue has been to quantify training loads (training demands) and a range of physiological and non-physiological parameters (responses to training). Quantifying training loads is more straightforward in individual sports, and user-created or commercially-available software is often used to capture, collate, analyse and report training data. In team sports, assessing training loads is more challenging given the diverse range of training activities commonly employed (e.g. general conditioning, resistance training, interval training and skill-based conditioning). Although the underlying physiological and psycho-physiological explanations for pacing, fatigue and regulation of exercise performance remain controversial [1-3], and require further investigation, it is clear that athletes, coaches and team personnel are seeking guidance on how to limit the negative aspects of fatigue on training and competitive performance.

Sport science evaluation of athletes has traditionally taken the form of routine (prospective) monitoring of physiological, non-physiological and performance measures. Routine testing generally involves measures taken at rest (baseline), and during and/or after laboratory testing, routine training or in competition settings [4]. Most sports scientists, coaches and athletes have experienced the traditional form of testing. Another approach is use of functional challenges (primarily administered in the laboratory or training settings) where athletes are exposed to repeated bouts of exercise to quantify responses and rates of recovery [5]. In many sports simple self-reported measures of well-being including fatigue, muscle soreness, patterns of sleep, mood state, quality of training, and resting heart rate, are used to monitor athletes [6]. The issue of social facilitation in team and individual sports relating to training loads, coping skills, and adaptive responses is also an important consideration. The issues of psychological and social factors, and their interaction with physiological processes and performance in the context of fatigue, require further multi-disciplinary research.

DEFINING FATIGUE

In a comprehensive scientific review of fatigue, St. Clair Gibson and colleagues [7] note that definitions of fatigue vary between fields of medicine, exercise physiology, neurophysiology and psychology. For example, most exercise physiologists recognise fatigue as, "... an acute impairment of exercise performance, which leads to an eventual inability to produce maximal force output as a consequence of metabolite accumulation or substrate depletion" [7]. With athletes, fatigue can be categorised by referencing the fatigue-inducing task (e.g., high frequency fatigue, eccentric contraction related fatigue, counter-movement jump fatigue, sustained endurance exercise fatigue). Fatigue can also be linked to the suspected anatomical location where the mechanism of fatigue is located [8, 9]. The term "central fatigue" refers to functional limitations originating from the brain, whereas peripheral fatigue is frequently used to describe the inability of a muscle to produce force due to perturbed intracellular environments such as glycogen depletion, hydrogen ion accumulation or an imbalance between intracellular sodium and potassium concentrations [10]. Although coaches and athletes may have a passing interest in mechanisms responsible for fatigue, most are more concerned with the magnitude, duration and consequences of fatigue on performance.

From a sport science perspective the *inability to complete a task that was once achievable within a recent time frame* is a practical definition of fatigue that coaches and athletes easily relate to. For instance, if an athlete's ability to perform pull ups is reduced from 20 to 10 following three sets of 15 pull-ups, then the reduced pull-up performance could be attributed to fatigue. In contrast, if an athlete was capable of 20 pull-ups two years ago but can only currently complete 15 pull-ups, fatigue is not necessarily the cause of the problem since the performance standard (20 pull-ups) was not achieved "within a recent time frame". In some cases, when an athlete fails to perform at an expected high standard, the athlete is not fatigued, but merely unfit, unwell, injured or unmotivated. It is also possible that adverse environmental conditions (e.g. heat, humidity, and altitude) are to blame for a lack-lustre performance. In these cases, it is inappropriate to assume fatigue was responsible for the less than personal best performance.

The magnitude of fatigue can often be quantified as a percent reduction in a standard performance task. For example, if an athlete can bench press 100kg but after a heavy week of training is only capable of lifting 80kg then the magnitude of fatigue is 20%. Assuming there was a similar "maximal effort" produced by the athlete before and after the heavy lifting, then residual fatigue in the execution of the bench press has been identified. The magnitude of fatigue is most likely task-specific. In the case of the bench press example, there could be a 20% reduction in the maximal mass that can be lifted but only a 10% reduction in the mass that can be lifted for 3 sets of 10 repetitions. Similarly, the average power output (i.e. a combination of contraction velocity and mass) for 2 lifts at 95kg might be reduced by 30% demonstrating how task specific the magnitude of fatigue may be. Techniques are now emerging that allow velocity-specific fatigue to be quantified during actual competition in international sprint cycling competition [11]. A sport-specific, contraction velocity-specific quantification of fatigue may provide insights into effective treatment and management approaches. Although conceptually quite simple, estimations of the magnitude of fatigue can quickly become complicated as it is often difficult to distinguish whether the explanation for an inadequate performance is a loss of fitness and/or accumulation of fatigue [12].

Initially, quantifying the duration of fatigue seems simple enough. After a heavy training phase or a particularly rigorous training session, an athlete could periodically attempt a standard performance task. The coach or scientist can then evaluate how long it takes before fatigue dissipates and performance reaches or exceeds a previous reference value. Fatigue lasting less than 24-48 hours is "short-term", whereas fatigue persisting for more than two days can be categorised as "long-term" fatigue. Unfortunately, using maximal performance tests to quantify magnitude and persistence of fatigue can introduce further fatigue [13]. Thus, the tests used to identify and quantify fatigue could confound the monitoring or understanding of the recovery process. Maximal performance tests can be difficult to perform consistently even when athletes are fresh and motivated. Consider the task of asking an extremely fatigued and irritable athlete to perform a maximal 1500m run every week following a very heavy 4 week training block. Longitudinal testing of maximal performance can be challenging in both logistic and psychological terms.

In response to the challenge of identifying fatigue in highly trained athletes, some researchers have developed submaximal tests in both laboratory and field settings. Heart Rate - Perception of Effort [14] and Lactate – Perception of Effort [15] indices at a given submaximal workload have been proposed as physiological indicators of fatigue. Tired athletes may have a reduced heart rate but an elevated rating of perceived exertion as they complete a graded exercise test. Similarly tired endurance athletes may display suppressed lactate levels but elevated perception of effort after rigorous training phases. Heavy training can influence these psycho – physiological indices but further work is required to establish how useful these ratios are for monitoring fatigue and guiding training loads in a manner that improves performance capabilities.

Fatigue can also be categorised retrospectively based on the performance outcome once the athlete is fully recovered from a block of heavy exercise. The consequences of fatigue can simplistically be categorised as "non-adaptive" or "adaptive" based on whether the athlete demonstrates a rebound in performance [16]. Distinguishing between heavy fatigue and inappropriate recovery can be a challenge, but assuming the athlete has followed contemporary recommendations for recovery (i.e., adequate nutrition and sleep, reduced training volume and adequate recovery duration between intense training sessions) it is possible to establish whether the fatigue-inducing training produced an "adaptive" or "non-adaptive" response. Numerous coaches have trained endurance athletes very hard for 2-3 weeks and then observed a poor performance at a competition following a 1-week taper. Surprisingly, there are examples of athletes who have recorded a personal best time 2-3 weeks after the disappointing result following one week of recovery. In this case, it would be inappropriate to categorise the fatigue as "non-adaptive" because the athlete responded to training; it just took longer than expected. Thus, the athlete mistimed the recovery process which is quite different from engaging in training that induces "non-adaptive" fatigue where there is no subsequent improvement in performance.

Many terms for fatigue have been published in the scientific literature including: overtraining, overreaching, unexplained underperformance, underperformance syndrome, fibromyalgia, chronic fatigue, persistent fatigue, non-functional over-reaching, functional over-reaching, tired, and burn out [9]. However, coaches and athletes tend to think about fatigue from a practical perspective. The magnitude (percent reduction in performance ability), duration (how long will performance impairment last) and nature of fatigue (adaptive fatigue refers to an improvement in performance following recovery whereas non-adaptive fatigue reflects no apparent improvement in performance following a heavy block of training) become important aspects of fatigue that can influence training programs. Researchers are currently working to establish physiological indicators that accurately reflect the severity of fatigue without requiring the athlete to perform a maximal physical challenge. At this stage, the best way to understand fatigue in an athlete may be to quantify their perceptions and sensations of fatigue as well as evaluate performance associated with "maximal" exertion [4, 7, 17, 18].

Team Sports

A key question in team sports research related to fatigue is the choice of dependent (outcome) measures. Traditionally this work has focused on the changes in physiological factors such as heart rate, blood lactate, sprint ability, or movement patterns quantified via time-motion analysis, or more recently global positioning system (GPS) tracking. The focus of future investigations will be on relationships between physiological factors, movement patterns and performance indicators. A fourth factor is the strategies and tactics employed by coaches to limit the effects of fatigue, or impose greater fatigue on opposition players and teams. It is apparent that social facilitation and psychosocial factors influence relationships between fatigue and performance in team sports. Some intriguing work in the fields of pain management [19] and wound healing [20] has shown important links between psychological and social factors and the time course for tissue repair. This line of investigation offers promise for management of fatigue in team sports from the perspective of both individual player and team performance.

In team sports, the most useful indicators of fatigue are decrements in performance, physiological measures and skill indicators. We conducted a study on the effects of fatigue on decision making and shooting skill-performance in water polo players to explore these relationships [21]. Fourteen junior elite male players completed four sets of eight maximal effort repetitions (~18 s per repetition) of a water polo-specific drill. A video-based temporally occluded decision making task or a goal shooting test was performed after each set. At very high levels of fatigue, decision-making accuracy was 18 ± 22% (mean ± 95% confidence limits) better than at low fatigue. Shooting accuracy and velocity were unaffected by fatigue, however skill proficiency (technique) decreased by 43 ± 24% after high-fatigue conditions. Incremental increases in fatigue differentially influenced decision making (improved) relative to the technical performance (declined), accuracy and speed of the ball (unchanged) of a water polo shot. These data indicate that fatigue can influence technical and performance tasks in different ways.

An imbalance between training loads and recovery can manifest as an increased risk of fatigue, injury and/or illness in team sport players depending on individual circumstances. Management of fatigue in team sports includes monitoring of the individual and team performance indicators, training loads, physiological and psychological measures, and psycho-physiological measures such as mood state, session rating of perceived exertion (RPE) and sport-specific questionnaires for athletes [22-24]. Although questionnaires are widely used, issues with validity, compliance and the degree the results are actually used to revise or modify training programs, often limit their usefulness. Short-term use of questionnaires is often more practical as athletes often tire of completing a daily questionnaire for long periods. The quality and timing of feedback for athletes is critical.

Individual Sports

In individual sports such as athletics, cycling, swimming, and triathlon, high training loads often leave athletes feeling fatigued. Management of fatigue centres primarily on careful prescription and periodisation of both short- and long-term training loads.

Periodisation of training remains an art as much as a science. The training programs adopted by elite athletes are commonly refined through trial and error over a period of time and are typically based on individual needs.

Training-induced fatigue concepts proposed in the 1980's by Dr. Eric Banister have influenced many endurance coaches and scientists in a variety of sports. Banister's ideas were both simple and intuitively appealing. In his early papers, Banister and co-workers presented performance as an outcome variable influenced by both fitness and fatigue [25]. Banister characterised fitness as a positive influence on performance that was slow to both develop and dissipate once training ceased. Fatigue on the other hand was characterised with a much shorter time constant reflecting a trait that could accumulate and dissipate quickly. These straight forward concepts seemed to reflect what many coaches were seeing in the field - heavy training was required for developing fitness and managing fatigue through recovery and prolonged tapers was essential to elicit quality performances. In Banister's model, fatigue can be assessed indirectly by accurately quantifying fitness linked to training load and performance. Sporting performance can be monitored reasonably accurately assuming consistent conditions and maximal effort. However, two challenges faced by those adopting Banister's model are how should training load be quantified and what time constants should be used for fitness and fatigue [12]. The training impulse (TRIMP) was initially proposed as the best indicator of training load. This load unit, similar to many other load units, is a combination of exercise duration and intensity [26]. Once daily training load is quantified it is then possible to mathematically evaluate the relationship between training load, performance and fatigue [12]. If an athlete's best performances are occurring much sooner after a loading block than the model predicts then it is possible to decrease the time constant for fatigue or essentially "tune" the model. Despite many iterations of the Banister model, coaches and athletes are only recently using software and the modelling approach to refine training management. Although creative and innovative training structures are a hallmark of the more successful training programs, simply giving more rest and recovery to athletes may be equally as important. Many different performance tests have evolved to monitor submaximal and maximal performance capacities in individual athletes [5]. There is ongoing debate on the merits of different exercise protocols that might be useful for diagnostic purposes.

To highlight some of issues in quantifying load we present an example in the sport of road cycling. Quantification of training load ranges from the simple (e.g. how many kilometres a cyclists rides) to the refined and complex (e.g. training impulse, sessional RPE and Training Stress Score™). The question often asked is, "What is the best way to quantify training load?" and most experienced sports scientists tend to reply, "It depends". The key question is what outcome measure the athlete or coach is interested in predicting or understanding. For those interested in injury quantifying a load unit that captures novel high tension loading has merit. Similarly, training volume, travel and emotional stress can increase the risk of illness. The ability to cope with heavy training loads (e.g. 1400km of riding per week) is best predicted by understanding progressions in training volume. In contrast, maximal power that can be produced for 4:15 min:sec (individual pursuit) is best understood by quantifying the amount of time the athlete produces high quality cycling power output (400-600W).

The advent of the portable heart rate monitor has been instrumental in establishing a number of "internal load" metrics including the Training Impulse defined by Banister and colleagues [25]. However, more recent advancements in miniaturised smart sensor technologies that allow movement speed and cycling power output to be quantified have increased interest in "external load" units. Cycling power output can now be converted to a Training Stress Score^{TM} (TSS^{TM}) by commercially available software. These load units are then used to understand patterns in training and predict periods when the athlete is likely to produce personal best performances. Only recently have researchers adopted the TSS^{TM} load unit which is based entirely on power output profiles produced during cycling as a unit of training load in scientific publications [27].

Many discussions and arguments have focused on whether internal load units are superior to external load units or vice versa. It may be the case that effective understanding of the athlete will come when both internal and external load units are monitored daily. The diagnostic relevance of monitoring two dimensions of training load appears to have merit. High power output (external load) with a low heart rate (internal load) may reflect a very different fatigue status than an athlete at the same power output but with a high heart rate. A combination of external and internal load units is probably required to reliably differentiate between fit and fresh vs. fit and tired.

Substantial efforts have been made to identify useful biomarkers for managing fatigue, health and performance of athletes [6, 28-30]. However, at present no single biomarker has sufficient sensitivity and specificity to effectively quantify the degree of acute and residual fatigue on a daily basis. Routine testing of biochemical, haematological, endocrinological and immunological parameters can be invasive and costly, and often yields little value in otherwise healthy individuals [31]. The search for gold standard biomarkers has proved elusive, and multivariate modelling is more likely to yield useful results than single measures alone [7, 9, 32]. However the time and expense of a multivariate approach is problematic for most sports. Both clinical/practical experience, and the results of observational and controlled experimental research, is needed to develop practical guidelines for managing fatigue in the field.

Historically, training sensations tend to be left in the realm of sport psychology. Recent research indicates that adaptations to training may be influenced by not only the internal and external load but the emotional state of the athlete when they engage in training [7, 33]. Quantification of training load may be refined and become more meaningful from a performance prediction perspective by understanding when an athlete is "hopeless" vs. "hopeful".

TRAINING PRESCRIPTION AND MANAGEMENT OF FATIGUE

While there are many studies on the acute effects of exercise and chronic effects of training the science of training prescription is less well described. Our experience with Australian athletes highlights the following key considerations: most individual and team sport athletes benefit from a well developed background of general fitness derived from volume-oriented training, small increments in training intensity and load limit the risk of short-term overreaching; shorter more frequent sessions are well tolerated by sprint-oriented athletes; skill-based conditioning is an effective way of developing both skills and fitness attributes; interval-based conditioning is the corner stone of developing high levels of fitness; nutrition and refuelling are important in supporting both training and competition; recovery practices need to be more comprehensive and aggressive with higher training loads, and short active off-seasons are recommended to limit detraining and fatigue at the commencement of the following season.

The increasing availability of funding and human resources, and emerging digital technology, is generating very large data sets in both team and individual sports. Sports-specific examples include data generated by SRM and power cranks in cycling, digital video of team sports, and the rapid expansion of GPS monitoring. In the past, most of the routine monitoring has been interpreted subjectively in the field, and more rigorous analysis has been left to experimental research of group data. However recent approaches have emerged for more detailed and meaningful evaluation of individual athlete data in a case study format. A systems-based approach that integrates well chosen diagnostic tests, with smart sensor technology, and a real-time database and data management system is the future for fatigue management. Practical/clinical significance with magnitude-based inferences and precision of estimation involving sports-specific reference or threshold values, observed changes or differences, typical error of measurement and a probabilistic approach, are emerging in the sports science literature [34, 35]. There are also approaches available to quantify the degree or magnitude of the (true) individual response to an intervention or fatigue that is free of measurement error [36]. A magnitude-based approach using sports-specific reference values yields valuable research insights, but also puts the results of routine athlete testing and controlled research in a more practical light for coaches, athletes and team personnel.

The management of fatigue centres on unloading the athlete, ensuring adequate rest, recovery and nutrition, application of various recovery interventions, and a graded return to full training. In most cases, athletes with short-term (acute) fatigue are ready to train at normal levels within 24-48 hours. In cases of more severe fatigue, a graded return involving a longer recovery period and sequential increases in training volume/duration, frequency, and intensity, is indicated. The time course of return to full training will depend on the severity and underlying cause(s) of fatigue. Premature resumption of full training can overload the athlete and lead to recurrence and/or persistence of fatigue. The most common recovery strategies include massage, stretching, compression garments, cryotherapy [37] , nutrition, aerobic exercise, and hydrotherapy [38]. Coaches of elite athletes recognise that the emotional state of the athlete may be equally as important as managing structural components of training and recovery. Perfect preparation isn't always going to lead to athletic success. However a carefully planned and executed training management strategy that minimises the effects of fatigue on training and competition should be a high priority for coaches and athletes. Researchers in sport science should welcome the opportunity to give careful and evidence-based advice for elite athletes as they prepare for important competition. The physical, psychological and nutritional influences that lead to truly exceptional performances are of interest to athletes, coaches and scientists.

References

[1] Tucker R, Noakes TD. The physiological regulation of pacing strategy during exercise: A critical review. *Br J Sports Med*, 2009, 43, 392-400.

[2] Tucker R. The anticipatory regulation of performance: The physiological basis for pacing strategies and the development of a perception-based model for exercise performance. *Br J Sports Med*, 2009, 43, 392-400.

[3] Shephard RJ. Is it time to retire the 'central governor'? *Sports Med*, 2009, 39, 709-21.

[4] Robson-Ansley PJ, Gleeson M, Ansley L. Fatigue management in the preparation of Olympic athletes. *J Sports Sci*, 2009, 27, 1409 -20

[5] Meeusen R, Nederhof E, Buyse L, Roelands B, Schutter GD, Piacentini MF. Diagnosing overtraining in athletes using the two bout exercise protocol. *Br J Sports Med*, 2008, 44, 642-8.

[6] Halson SL, Jeukendrup AE. Does overtraining exist? An analysis of overreaching and overtraining research. *Sports Med*, 2004, 34, 967-81.

[7] St Clair Gibson A, Baden DA, Lambert MI, Lambert EV, Harley YX, Hampson D, et al. The conscious perception of the sensation of fatigue. *Sports Med*, 2003, 33, 167-76.

[8] Kuipers H. Training and overtraining: an introduction. *Med Sci Sports Exerc*, 1998, 30, 1137-9.

[9] Uusitalo AL. Overtraining: Making a difficult diagnosis and implementing targeted treatment. *Phys Sportsmed*, 2001, 29, 35-50.

[10] Meeusen R, Watson P, Hasegawa H, Roelands B, Piacentini MF. Brain neurotransmitters in fatigue and overtraining. *Appl Physiol Nutr Metab*, 2007, 32, 857-64.

[11] Gardner AS, Martin DT, Jenkins DG, Dyer I, Van Eiden J, Barras M, et al. Velocity-specific fatigue: Quantifying fatigue during variable velocity cycling. *Med Sci Sports Exerc*, 2009, 41, 904-11.

[12] Morton RH. Modeling training and overtraining. *J Sports Sci*, 1997, 15, 335-40.

[13] Kuipers H, Keizer HA. Overtraining in elite athletes: Review and directions for the future. *Sports Med*, 1988, 6, 79-92.

[14] Martin DT, Andersen MB. Heart rate-perceived exertion relationship during training and taper. *J Sports Med Phys Fitness*, 2000, 40, 201-8.

[15] Snyder AC, Jeukendrup AE, Hesselink MK, Kuipers H, Foster C. A physiological/psychological indicator of over-reaching during intensive training. *Int J Sports Med*, 1993, 14, 29-32.

[16] Budgett R. Fatigue and underperformance in athletes: The overtraining syndrome. *Br J Sports Med*, 1998, 32, 107-10.

[17] Angeli A, Minetto M, Dovio A, Paccotti P. The overtraining syndrome in athletes: A stress-related disorder. *J Endocrinol Invest*, 2004, 27, 603-12.

[18] Roose J, de Vries WR, Schmikli SL, Backx FJ, van Doornen LJ. Evaluation and opportunities in overtraining approaches. *Res Q Exerc Sport*, 2009, 80, 756-64.

[19] Finestone HM, Alfeeli A, Fisher WA. Stress-induced physiologic changes as a basis for the biopsychosocial model of chronic musculoskeletal pain: A new theory? *Clin J Pain*, 2008, 24, 767-75.

[20] Detillion CE, Craft TKS, Glasper ER, Prendergast BJ, DeVries AC. Social facilitation of wound healing. *Pyschoneuroendocrinology*, 2004, 29, 1004-11.

[21] Royal KA, Farrow D, Mujika I, Halson SL, Pyne D, Abernethy B. The effects of fatigue on decision making and shooting skill performance in water polo players. *J Sports Sci*, 2006, 24, 807-15.

[22] Fitzpatrick MW, Robertson RJ, Powers JM, Mears JL, Ferrer NF. Comparisons of RPE before, during and after self-regulated aerobic exercise. *Med Sci Sports Exerc*, 2009, 41, 682-7.

[23] Borresen J, Lambert MI. Quantifying training load: A comparison of subjective and objective methods. *Int J Sports Physiol Per*, 2008, 3, 16-30.

[24] Alexiou H, Coutts A. A comparison of methods used for quantifying internal training load in women soccer players. *Int J Sports Physiol Per*, 2008, 3, 320-30.

[25] Banister EW, Calvert TW. Planning for future performance: Implications for long term training. *Can J Appl Sport Sci*, 1980, 5, 170-6.

[26] Morton RH, Fitz-Clarke JR, Banister EW. Modeling human performance in running. *J Appl Physiol*, 1990, 69, 1171-7.

[27] Garvican LA, Martin DT, McDonald W, Gore CJ. Seasonal variation of haemoglobin mass in internationally competitive female road cyclists. *Eur J Appl Physiol*, 2010, 109, 221-31.

[28] Hartmann U, Mester J. Training and overtraining markers in selected sport events. *Med Sci Sports Exerc*, 2000, 32, 209-15.

[29] Hawley CJ, Schoene RB. Overtraining syndrome: A guide to diagnosis, treatment, and prevention. *Phys Sportsmed*, 2003, 31, 25-31.

[30] St Clair Gibson A, Grobler LA, Collins M, Lambert MI, Sharwood K, Derman EW, et al. Evaluation of maximal exercise performance, fatigue, and depression in athletes with acquired chronic training intolerance. *Clin J Sport Med*, 2006, 16, 39-45.

[31] Fallon KE. The clinical utility of screening of biochemical parameters in elite athletes: Analysis of 100 cases. *Br J Sports Med*, 2008, 42, 334-7.

[32] Petibois C, Cazorla G, Poortmans JR, Deleris G. Biochemical aspects of overtraining in endurance sports: A review. *Sports Med*, 2002, 32, 867-78.

[33] Baron B, Moullan F, Deruelle F, Noakes TD. The role of emotions on pacing strategies and performance in middle and long duration sport events. *Br J Sports Med*, 2010, [Epub ahead of print] June 17.

[34] Batterham A, Hopkins WG. Making meaningful inferences about magnitudes. *Int J Sports Physiol Per*, 2006, 1, 50-7.

[35] Hopkins WG, Batterham A, Marshall SW, Hanin J. Progressive statistics for studies in sports medicine and exercise science. *Med Sci Sports Exerc*, 2009, 41, 3-13.

[36] Pyne D, Hopkins WG, Batterham A, Gleeson M, Fricker PA. Characterising the individual performance responses to mild illness in international swimmers. *Br J Sports Med*, 2005, 39, 752-6.

[37] Vaile J, Halson S, Gill N, Dawson B. Effect of cold water immersion on repeat cycling performance and thermoregulation in the heat. *J Sports Sci*, 2008, 26, 431-40.

[38] Vaile J, Halson S, Dawson B. Effect of hydrotherapy on recovery from fatigue. *Int J Sports Med*, 2008, 29, 539-44.

INDEX

B

C

D

E

F

G

H

I

J

K

L

M

N

O

P

Q

R

T

U

V

W

Y